Palliative and End of Life Care for Paramedics

Disclaimer

Class Professional Publishing have made every effort to ensure that the information, tables, drawings and diagrams contained in this book are accurate at the time of publication. The book cannot always contain all the information necessary for determining appropriate care and cannot address all individual situations; therefore, individuals using the book must ensure they have the appropriate knowledge and skills to enable suitable interpretation. Class Professional Publishing does not guarantee, and accepts no legal liability of whatever nature arising from or connected to, the accuracy, reliability, currency or completeness of the content of Palliative and End of Life Care for Paramedics. Users must always be aware that such innovations or alterations after the date of publication may not be incorporated in the content. Please note, however, that Class Professional Publishing assumes no responsibility whatsoever for the content of external resources in the text or accompanying online materials.

The information presented in this book is accurate and current to the best of the authors' knowledge.

The authors and publisher, however, make no guarantee as to, and assume no responsibility for, the correctness, sufficiency or completeness of such information or recommendation.

Printing history
This edition first published 2020

The authors and publisher welcome feedback from the users of this book. Please contact the publisher:

Class Professional Publishing,

The Exchange, Express Park, Bristol Road, Bridgwater TA6 4RR

Telephone: 01278 472 800

Email: post@class.co.uk

Website: www.classprofessional.co.uk

Class Professional Publishing is an imprint of Class Publishing Ltd

A CIP catalogue record for this book is available from the British Library

Paperback ISBN: 9781859596715

eBook ISBN: 9781859596722

Cover design by Hybert Design Limited, UK
Designed and typeset by S4Carlisle Publishing Services
Printed in the UK by Cambrian Printers Ltd

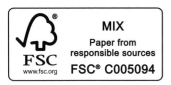

Refer to local recycling guidance on disposal of this book.

Contents

Contents

Contents

Disclaimer

The details in this book are presented for information purposes only. Paramedics and healthcare professionals should always follow local procedures and be aware of their own scope of practice.

Acknowledgements

I would like to thank my husband David, daughters Phillipa and Dorothea, brother Mark, cousin Lisa and friends Caroline, Corinne, Martin and Paula for their unwavering faith in me. Also, Dr Tim Clark for his continuing mentorship. Without their support this book would have not been completed.

In addition, I would like to thank the book's inspiring contributors, Alison, Fiona, Kath, Lindsay, Marlon and Stephen, for sharing their invaluable knowledge and expertise. I would also like to thank Professor Karen Cleaver for her kind and gracious words in the Foreword.

My deepest thanks and gratitude to you all.

Tania Blackmore

Abbreviations and Acronyms

5-HT	serotonin
ABC	airway, breathing, circulation
ABCD	airway, breathing, circulation, disability
ACP	advance care plan
AD	advance directive
ADRT	advance decision to refuse specified treatment
BD	*bis in die* (l.) twice daily
COPD	chronic obstructive pulmonary disease
CPR	cardiopulmonary resuscitation
CRP	C-reactive protein
CSCI	continuous subcutaneous infusion
CT	computed tomography
CTZ	chemotactic trigger zone
DNACPR	do not attempt cardiopulmonary resuscitation
ECG	electrocardiogram
eGFR	estimated glomerular filtration rate
EMS	emergency medical services
EOLCS	End of Life Care Strategy
FEARS	fears, environment, attitudes, responses, skills
FIBS	fears, inadequate skills, beliefs, support
GCS	Glasgow Coma Scale
GI	Gastrointestinal
GMC	General Medical Council
GSF	Gold Standards Framework
HCPC	Health and Care Professions Council
IAHPC	International Association for Hospice and Palliative Care
IHCD	institute for Healthcare Development
IM	intramuscular
INR	international normalized ratio
IR	instant-release
IV	intravenous
LACDP	Leadership Alliance for the Care of Dying People

LCP	Liverpool Care Pathway
LPA	lasting power of attorney
MASCC	Multinational Association for Supportive Care in Cancer
MCA	mental capacity act
MR	modified-release
MSCC	metastatic spinal cord compression
NICE	National Institute for Health and Care Excellence
NMC	Nursing and Midwifery Council
NRS	noisy respiratory secretions
NSAIDs	non-steroidal anti-inflammatory drugs
PCT	primary care trust
PO	per os (oral administration)
POT	palliative oxygen therapy
PRN	pro re nata
PTSD	post-traumatic stress disorder
QAA	Quality Assurance Agency
ReSPECT	Recommended Summary Plan for Emergency Care and Treatment
RT	radiotherapy
SACT	systemic anti-cancer treatment
SBRT	stereotactic body radiation therapy
SC	subcutaneous
SNRIs	serotonin and noradrenaline reuptake inhibitors
SQUiD	Single Question in Delirium
SSRIs	selective serotonin reuptake inhibitors
SVCS	superior vena cava syndrome
SVC	superior vena cava
WHO	World Health Organization

About the Authors

Tania Blackmore is a Senior Lecturer in Palliative and End of Life Care in the Faculty of Education, Health and Human Sciences at the University of Greenwich. Tania completed her nurse training at Charing Cross School of Nursing, London in 1988 working in trauma and orthopaedics before specialising in HIV and AIDS. In the late eighties and early nineties, she worked at The World's End Health Centre, The Thomas Macaulay Unit at St Stephen's and Westminster Hospital and at the Kobler Centre Chelsea specialising in AIDS as well as working on drug trials studying combinations to fight HIV. In 2014, after many years working in the community, hospice and acute sector as a Clinical Nurse Specialist in palliative care, Tania completed her MSc in Advance Practice in Palliative Care at Canterbury Christ Church University, gaining a distinction for her research project which explored acute clinicians' views on caring for palliative patients. She is also a Fellow of the Higher Education Academy (FHEA). Tania is responsible for delivering all aspects of palliative and end of life education across the paramedic programme such as symptom control, breaking bad news, ethical and legal aspects of death, bereavement, loss, grief and professional resilience. Tania is currently studying for her PhD at the International Observatory on End of Life Care, at Lancaster University. Her research is focused on parental loss in families with young children.

Stephen Cox is a Visiting Professor in the Faculty of Social and Life Sciences at Glyndŵr University, Wrexham. An interest in medicine developed during research work on the geography of mental illness and he went on to study medicine in Southampton with postgraduate studies in Oxford. Stephen's interest in the overlap between medicine and geography culminated in an attachment to the MRC Environmental Epidemiology Unit studying the geography of thyroid disease in Stoke on Trent. During postgraduate training he worked at Sobell House Hospice in Oxford at a time when palliative care was beginning to emerge as a distinct specialty. After a twenty-year career in both general practice and a role as team doctor to a professional football club, he returned to hospice medicine at Pilgrims Hospices in East Kent. In addition to clinical work he was Principal Investigator for studies on prognostication and hydration at end of life.

Lindsay Hart is a Clinical Education Facilitator at the University of Greenwich. She is a registered paramedic and has held roles within the ambulance service which have included Clinical Team Leader and Community Paramedic, which concentrated predominantly on urgent and primary care. Lindsay has a Master's degree in Education and teaches across a variety of modules at the university, mainly focusing on the BSc (Hons) Paramedic Science Degree programme. She has a keen interest in paramedic education around end of life and palliative care, along with exploring the resilience and wellbeing of both student paramedics and qualified ambulance clinicians.

Kath Jennings is the Academic Lead for Paramedic Science and leader of undergraduate paramedic programmes at the University of Greenwich. In her role she provides leadership of teaching and scholarly activity within the Faculty of Education, Health and Human Sciences. Her clinical experience was gained while working for the London Ambulance Service NHS Trust as an emergency medical technician and a paramedic. Her teaching interest began in the further education sector after graduating from her first degree. As a paramedic, Kath has been a lecturer/senior lecturer at the University of Hertfordshire and at the University of Greenwich. She acquired her MA in Education in 2015 and is currently undertaking doctoral studies in the field of paramedic education. Her research interests and publications to date include paramedic management of pelvic injuries, paramedic students' understanding of emotional labour in paramedic practice, interprofessional education and leadership for paramedics.

Fiona Kiely is a Consultant in Palliative Medicine at Marymount University Hospital and Hospice, Cork, Ireland and Senior Clinical Lecturer, University College Cork, Ireland, her alma mater. She leads interdisciplinary teams in the care of patients with complex palliative care needs in the community, acute hospitals and a 44-bed specialist palliative care inpatient unit located in Cork. She is also currently studying for her PhD at the Division of Health Research, Lancaster University. Her research is focused on extended survivorship in advanced cancers. Fiona is dual qualified as a general practitioner and holds diplomas in Medicine of the Elderly, Child Health, Clinical Psychiatry and Clinical Dermatology awarded by the Royal College of Physicians in Ireland, the Royal College of Surgeons in Ireland and Cardiff University. Additional postgraduate scholarships have included a clinical observership in the Harvard Medical School- affiliated Brigham and Women's Hospital, Boston, Massachusetts, as well as clinical experience in Princess Alexandra Hospital, Brisbane, Australia. She currently chairs the research committee in Marymount University Hospital and Hospice and personal research interests and publications include topics such as early integration of palliative care, information transfer out-of-hours for community palliative care patients, structured outcome measurement in palliative care and the use of big data and technology to support the delivery of specialist palliative care.

Alison Rae is a Senior Lecturer in Adult Nursing and Paramedic Science at the University of Greenwich. With an acute care background in adult nursing, she has worked in a variety of clinical settings including gynaecology/oncology, accident and emergency, resuscitation training (including advanced life support and generic instructor training), site management and surgical assessment. She left the NHS after 20 years in practice to pursue a career in academia where she is now responsible for overseeing the delivery of several pre- and post-registration courses, including the leadership in practice module for the BSc Paramedic Science programme. With a Master's in Advanced Practice, she has an interest in developing autonomous practice and improving enhanced clinical practice and interprofessional collaboration across all disciplines.

Marlon Stiell is a Senior Lecturer at the University of Greenwich where he is responsible for teaching law and ethics and research methods to undergraduate paramedic science students. He worked for the London Ambulance Service between 1994 and 2014, initially as a paramedic and then as an emergency care practitioner. He graduated with a BSc in Psychology in 2009 and completed his MSc in Health Psychology in 2013. His research interests are health psychology, ethics and dementia care.

Foreword

I am delighted to have been asked to write the foreword to this book. As a nurse with a clinical and academic background in emergency care, I have witnessed the transformation of the paramedic role from those required to transport critically ill (and indeed, not so unwell) patients, to a role that now requires a high level of clinical expertise. This transformation has included role redesign with the introduction of advanced roles including paramedic practitioners and emergency care practitioners. Both these roles aim to avoid transportation to overcrowded hospital emergency departments, providing patient care at home or closer to home instead.

There is generally a view that people would prefer to die at home; indeed, research indicates that the number of people dying at home or in care homes is increasing and by 2040 is predicted to further increase by 88.6% and 108.1% respectively (Bone et al., 2017). This increase in death outside of hospital in the UK is reflected in the experiences of paramedics, with a third of paramedics reporting that they attend to a terminally ill patient on each shift and a further 29% every other shift (Munday et al., 2011). It is evident therefore that providing end of life care has become, and will increasingly be, an integral element of the paramedic role and skill set. However, as Tania Blackmore notes in the opening chapter to this book, death and dying remain taboo areas of society which are often hidden and feared. Tania highlights how the use of language and euphemisms to describe death or impending death reflects the fear of explicitly talking about death and dying.

The historical emphasis within paramedic training to ensure adequate preparedness for managing acute trauma, medical and surgical emergencies has meant that end of life care has to date received comparatively little attention. Death is at odds with the aims and purpose of biomedicine. It is, therefore, no surprise to find that paramedics feel that they are inadequately prepared to care for patients who are at the end of their life (Kirk et al., 2017), and while confidence develops with experience, there is widespread agreement that paramedics require more training to improve their knowledge and practice around end of life care, thus this book is hugely timely.

Research undertaken in Australia which described the incidence and reason for attendance by paramedics for patients with a history of palliative care identified that the most common paramedic assessments were 'respiratory' (20.1%), 'pain' (15.8%) and 'deceased' (7.9%) (Lord et al., 2019). Tania Blackmore and her colleagues have addressed each of these areas in detail within the book.

The book follows a logical journey starting out with the broader historical, social and cultural debates about death and dying, and then goes on to explain in detail what palliative care entails and the policy background to current palliative care practice in the UK. The book then moves on to specific aspects of palliative care in paramedic practice giving a very informative overview of palliative care emergencies and how to recognise them. This is followed by a chapter on symptom management which likewise provides handy hints and explanations for the specific symptoms associated with terminal illness. This chapter provides accessible descriptions of symptoms, and detailed information on how these should be managed, with reference to a range of supporting literature, both in this chapter and indeed throughout the book. The next chapter then explores and discusses the broader skill sets associated with palliative care, including enhanced communication skills and caring for the dying patient, with an excellent overview of medication management at the end of life as well as discussion about what constitutes a 'good death'. Tania's chapter on care of the dying patient and her description of delirium and how to manage this is particularly welcome as this is an especially distressing condition for those who are dying and those witnessing death. Ethical principles underpinning paramedic practice with the dying patient, professional resilience and the paramedic's role as an end of life specialist complete the book, drawing together a rounded, encompassing and authoritative resource to aid paramedics in their everyday practice as well as academic based work. The case studies provided are particularly useful and offer an excellent resource for paramedic educators as well as students.

Tania and her co-writers have produced an accessible and highly informative book which I am sure will be an invaluable resource for paramedics and, indeed, other healthcare professionals. The book is a welcome addition to the growing academic resource and evidence base for paramedic science.

Karen Cleaver

References

Bone AE et al. (2017). What is the impact of population ageing on the future provision of end-of-life care? Population-based projections of place of death. *Palliative Medicine*, 32(2): 329–336.

Kirk A et al. (2017). Paramedics and their role in end-of-life care: perceptions and confidence. *Journal of Paramedic Practice,* 9: 71–79.

Lord B et al. (2019). Palliative care in paramedic practice: a retrospective cohort study. *Palliative Medicine*, 33(4): 445–51.

Munday D, Gakhal S, Bronnert R (2011). End-of-life care (EoLC) and emergency ambulance clinicians in the UK: reported practices in clinical management and views on Do Not Resuscitate orders (DNAR). 12th Congress of the European Association for Palliative Care, Lisbon, Portugal.

Chapter 1

Death and Dying in Society

Tania Blackmore

Introduction

Discussion of death and dying is shunned in our society, both in normal daily life and surprisingly also in clinical practice. In order to understand how health systems deal with the care of the dying, it is not enough just to base our understanding on the available numerical evidence. We, as clinicians, also need to appreciate the historical viewpoint; the philosophy behind our perceptions of human mortality, modern cure-targeted medicine and our changing lifestyles (Corr, 2016). The way that society perceives death is vital, as these attitudes determine the provisions and policies which are put into place for caring for those at the end of life. A recent systematic review calling for further research into public attitudes highlights this (Cox et al., 2013). To explore what underpins our collective cultural perspective towards incurable disease and care of the dying this chapter will discuss the following:

- Death in the pre-modern era
- Death in the modern era
- The effect of the biomedical model on clinical practice
- Clinical language used in palliative and end of life care
- The biopsychosocial model
- The need for holistic assessment in paramedic practice.

Death in the Pre-Modern Era

In pre-modern society, communities were made up of close extended families living in small compact dwellings, so death was seen in everyday life and learnt about by direct observation of the dying process (Walter, 2017b). Death in the pre-modern era was a communal event that took place in the home while the dying were cared for entirely by their families (Nebel Pederson and Emmers-Sommer, 2012). Death was presided over by the church, with the priest seen as the authoritative figure. Life expectancy was low (the average life expectancy between 1276 and 1300 being only 31.3 years, for example) and child mortality rates were high; as such, death was highly visible in society.

As society progressed into the twelfth century, death was seen in more individualistic terms with people beginning to consider how their own death might happen (Ariès, 1974). Life expectancy was on the increase and by the thirteenth century you could hope to live to 45 years of age and, statistically, if you had made it to your thirties, you might even have made it to your fifties. Death was increasingly dramatised and romanticised between the twelfth and eighteenth centuries, as evidenced by its increased depiction in art and in religious artefacts on tombs, which resulted in what Ariès describes as an 'exaggeration' of death by the nineteenth century (Ariès, 1974). This romanticising of death can be seen in Victorian death culture, with Victorians wearing brooches containing locks of hair from deceased loved ones (Figure 1.1) and the idealistic descriptions of death in literature by Brontë, Hardy and Rossetti (Lutz, 2011). It was not abnormal in the Victorian era to photograph your dead loved one and keep this photograph of them on the mantlepiece alongside images of them when they were alive (Figure 1.2).

> ## *Pause for thought*
>
> Owning a collection of mourning brooches may seem a little morbid, but they can be a surprisingly useful teaching aid when discussing attitudes towards death in palliative care lectures. Theses brooches demonstrate the Victorians' romanticising of death. Looking at the brooches like this evokes surprising discussions within the classroom as it gives the students a chance to ask questions about dying and death that they may find difficult to ask in the larger lecture group. If you look carefully you can see the different shades of hair in this brooch!

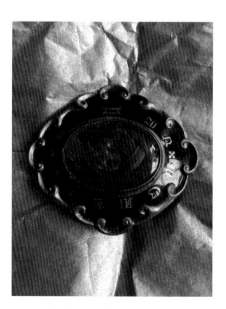

Figure 1.1   Example of a mourning brooch containing a lock of hair from the deceased
Source: Author's own collection

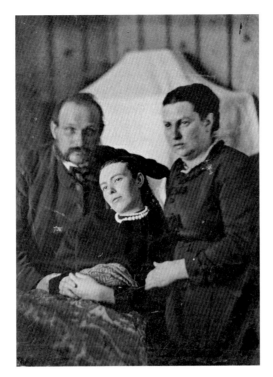

Figure 1.2   An example of Victorian post-mortem photography
Source: Private collection

Death in the Modern Era

Death has changed in the modern era – epidemics that affected past generations, such as influenza, typhus, the plague, smallpox, bacterial infections and some cancers, no longer have the same impact. Vaccinations, chemotherapy and antibiotics have eradicated many illnesses and as a result an ageing population is on the rise in western Europe and America (Kübler-Ross, 1970). There is an academic view that, because so many illnesses can be cured by medical and scientific advances, western society has assumed a culture of 'death denying' (Zimmermann and Rodin, 2004) and although logically death is an unavoidable part of clinical practice, it continues to be a neglected issue in our modern healthcare system because of our cultural collective death-denying coping mechanism (Thulesius et al., 2013).

We are now in a historical period where death and dying is rationalised while advancements in science and medicine mean that death no longer occurs in the home, but more predominantly in the hospital setting. In the hospital setting there is a great emphasis on cure which means that dying is often seen as a medical problem which can be overcome through medicine (Nebel Pederson and Emmers-Sommer, 2012). As a consequence, in modern times, death and dying is more likely to occur unwitnessed and in an institution. Often illness has many different disease trajectories because of a plethora of available medical interventions (Walter, 2017b).

The medicalisation of death in our modern society is seen by some to have led to a fear of the discussion of death and dying, and according to Ariès (1974), death is no longer acceptable in our modern society and as such needs to be hidden away in hospital and disguised by funeral directors. Alongside Ariès (1974), the philosopher Ernest Becker (1973) explored the description of western societies as being 'death denying', and the culture within these societies enforcing the practice of the hiding of death from the normal human experience (Sayer, 2010). Ariès (1974) described how modern western societies saw death as 'shameful and forbidden' and not to be acknowledged or discussed for fear that it would upset the normal status of regular life (Zimmermann and Rodin, 2004). Ariès's book, although written in the mid 1970s, is still relevant towards our understanding of how modern society views death and dying. The book was based on a series of lectures Ariès gave in the United States describing western attitudes to death from the middle ages to modern times (Ariès, 1974). There is a vivid description in the book of how death and dying is directly interpreted by society in line with scientific, industrial and religious changes. Becker's 1973 book, *The Denial of Death*, describes modern attitudes to death in psychoanalytic and theological terms in an attempt to understand our 'terror of death' (Becker, 1973: 11). Becker suggests that we are not born with a fear of death but acquire this fear as part of our psychological growth from childhood to adulthood, reinforced by the norms of our society.

The prevalence of a lack of discussion of death is the norm in wider general society as well as in clinical practice and the ever-evolving sphere of medicine. The medicalisation of death is perpetuated by us, the clinicians, as we are intent on prolonging or avoiding death as our main goal of treatment in clinical intervention with a subconscious need to eradicate death all together (Zimmermann and Rodin, 2004). Death in modern culture is now perceived as a scientific problem (Yurevich, 2018) rather than a natural occurrence. There is a philosophical viewpoint that you can assess the values and characteristics of a particular society by its collective attitudes to death and dying (Yurevich, 2018). If this is the case, perhaps we should reflect on why British hospices are mainly funded by the charity sector and why most people still die within institutions as opposed to their own home.

The medicalisation of death is just one of the themes seen in the study of death and dying in modern society. There are an accepted set of procedures and perspectives in death and dying that occur as part of how modern society deals with death (McManus, 2012), and these are:

- The medicalisation of death
- The institutionalisation of death
- The professionalisation of undertakers
- The commodification of funerals
- The secularisation of funerals

- The industrialisation of the disposal of the body
- The psychologising of death, grief and loss.

(McManus, 2012)

The components of death in the modern era are processes that occur away from the community by the medicalisation of death, death as an industry and death as a commercial commodity. The differences between death in the pre-modern era versus death in the modern era are summarised in Table 1.1.

Table 1.1 Differences in the cultural aspects of death and dying – pre-modern versus modern.

Pre-Modern Era	Modern Era
Frame of religion	Frame of reason
Religious ritual	Social ritual
Religious event	Medical event
Dying at home	Dying in hospital
Rooted in community	Private
Priest, authority	Doctor, authority
Age expectancy, low	Age expectancy, up
Death part of life	Taboo/denial

(Adapted from Walter, 1994)

Funeral Poverty

The funeral in modern Britain is no longer a religious ritual – it has become a service where we hand over the body of our loved ones as soon as possible to a one-stop funeral director who arranges the ceremony, music and disposal of the body (Walter, 2017a). The average cost of a basic burial in the UK in 2018 was £4,561, while a cremation was £3,596; the additional legal fees took the average cost of dying in the UK in 2018 up to £9,394. This represents an overall increase in funeral expenses of 4.7% since 2017 alone. This increasing cost has led to the term 'funeral poverty', with one in five families struggling to pay for their loved one's funeral (SunLife, 2018). Walter (2017a) suggests that the commercialisation of death may see a backlash from grieving families, whereby in the future funerals will go back to individuals in the community conducting their own funerals for their loved ones, not just in an attempt to cut costs, but to ensure that funerals are more personalised and that the deceased are cared for to the end, not made a component or a product of a huge industry.

The Effect of the Biomedical Model and Death Denial on Clinical Practice

The medicalisation of death is closely associated with the biomedical model approach to healthcare, the biomedical model of care being where the main emphasis of medical intervention is based on cure of patients, while death is perceived as an enemy that science and medicine can defeat (Nebel Pederson and Emmers-Sommer, 2012). While we would like the clinician looking after us to be intent on our cure and recovery, there has to be an acknowledgement in medical practice of the fact that we are all mortal. We cannot escape as human beings the undeniable reality that we are all going to die. In the words of Becker, 'the idea of death, the fear of it, haunts the human animal like nothing else; it is a mainspring of human activity – activity designed largely to avoid the fatality of death, to overcome it by denying in some way that it is the final destination of man' (1973: xvii).

The biomedical model looks at death as something to be conquered but, if encountered, it should be dealt with via two major approaches: (1) the verification of death, and (2) the cause of death (McManus, 2012). These two approaches lead to a culture that does not embrace care of the dying or an acceptance of death as part of the end of the life continuum in our healthcare system. Recent research suggests that modern healthcare should veer away from the biomedical model with its false death-denying promises and seeming surfeit of life-prolonging interventions at any cost (Llewellyn et al., 2016).

Clinical Language Used in Palliative and End of Life Care

A good example of how the biomedical model prevails in modern medicine is examined in how healthcare professionals use language to described dying in the acute health sector. A study by Wentlandt et al. (2018) examined the prevalence of ambiguous and euphemistic language to describe the dying and deaths of patients. The use of such language underpins the avoidance and non-acceptance of death in acute medicine. The following are unclear themes of language which are often used to describe the dying process:

- High mortality risk
- Situation is potentially a terminal event
- Grave situation
- Doing poorly
- Irreversible state
- Patient is comfort measures only
- New developments in prognosis
- Prognosis guarded

- Worsening overall prognosis
- Palliative philosophy of care.

(Wentlandt et al., 2018)

As clinicians we must be direct in our language when discussing death and dying, using direct terms such as 'dying', 'death' and 'dead', and stopping the use of euphemisms. By using terms such as 'passing away', 'unsuccessful resuscitation', 'at peace' or 'departed' in our attempts as clinicians to soften the impact on our patients and their loved ones, we only achieve confusion and misunderstanding. The Wentlandt et al. (2018) study enforces that the clinician's discomfort in discussing death and dying can cause distressing miscommunication between different healthcare professionals, but more importantly, further research indicates that not using direct terms such as death and dying may cause the patients and their loved ones to miss chances to spend precious time together (Kelemen and Groninger, 2018). The speciality of palliative and end of life care is not free from the use of euphemism: when we ask patients about their preferred place of care at end of life, are we not in fact asking 'preferred place of death' (Agar et al., 2008)? As clinicians we must be clear on how we communicate: this is discussed by Alison Rae in Chapter 5 – Enhanced Communication Skills in Palliative and End of Life Care.

An example of this comes from Southern Australia. A very newly qualified nurse from the UK who was working in a country hospital was told 'bed four has gone into town'. This caused much hilarity in a ward meeting among the staff when they asked if the patient had self-discharged – 'gone into town' being a euphemism for having died. The country hospital was in the bush and the nearest town was two hours away; you went there for groceries or to be buried.

The Biopsychosocial Model

The biomedical model is used predominantly within the acute sector in healthcare, a model underpinned by anatomy and physiology of disease as the fundamental factor of how clinicians treat patients. It has been suggested that adopting a biopsychosocial model of care for patients in primary care in the community is more congruent with achieving the best patient outcomes and effective treatment. The biopsychosocial model in clinical practice looks at disease as a blend of not only biological symptoms but also psychological and social components (Figure 1.3) that are attributed to the manifestation of disease and, as such, the clinician in primary care not only needs to offer a scientific approach to care, but also empathy and compassion to achieve the best patient outcomes (Kusnanto et al., 2018). The biopsychosocial model was originally outlined by Georg Engels in his 1977 research article describing the dangers of clinical practice's reliance on the biomedical model as an explanation of the trajectory of illness and its treatment (Wade and Halligan, 2017). It has been said that the biopsychosocial model is not the only perspective

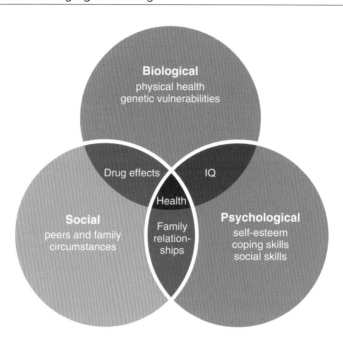

Figure 1.3 The biopsychosocial model of health

that can be used as an alternative to the rigid and one-dimensional view of the biomedical model, as there are other models such as the social model, but on the whole, research focuses on the biopsychosocial model as the alternative to the biomedical model (Wade and Halligan, 2017). Research also suggests that each of the three domains in each circle should be treated by the clinician equally (Jull, 2017).

There is a need to understand the components of the biopsychosocial model to understand the principles of palliative and end of life care. As previously discussed, the biomedical model, which is focused on cure and a death-denying philosophy, is not applicable to the care of incurable and dying patients. We need a health system that understands the values of providing effective care for the individual, and this needs a model that sees not only illness from the clinician's perspective but also the needs of the patient through providing a patient-centred approach. When a patient receives an incurable prognosis within the biomedical care approach, the clinical response to this patient is often an attitude of 'there is nothing more that medicine can do for them', which can lead to a feeling of abandonment, whereas the biopsychosocial model acknowledges the health professional's role in providing holistic care that addresses the patient's continuing need for physical, psychological and social support (Khoo Siew, 2005). There is a need within paramedic practice to use a holistic approach to the assessment of patients in order to provide good quality care for an ageing population with chronic and palliative healthcare needs (O'Meara et al., 2017). If there is acknowledgement and education within paramedic practice of the psychosocial factors of deterioration in the care of dying patients, this would be instrumental in achieving patient-centred care for palliative patients (Swetenham et al., 2014).

Conclusion

The research suggests that in order for ambulance clinicians to achieve a holistic assessment of palliative and end of life patients in their care, they need to have received education in the following subjects and concepts:

- Do not attempt cardiopulmonary resuscitation (DNACPR) decisions and documentation.
- Whether to transfer patients at end of life to hospice or hospital.
- Knowledge of how to access and refer patients to a specialist while the ambulance clinicians are in the patient's home.
- An awareness and understanding of advance directives and advance care planning documentation.
- Enhanced communication skills with patients, their loved ones and relatives.
- An understanding of symptom control, especially pain control.

(Adapted from Pettifer and Bronnert, 2013)

These education needs are the fundamental concepts of the principles of palliative and end of life care, which will be discussed fully in this textbook.

Pause for thought

To illustrate the use of death and dying euphemisms in the general population, list as many words and phrases for death and dying as you can think of. This might seem like a simple exercise but it's a good way of thinking about how we view death in society in the UK.

The brevity of phrases used to signify death highlights the importance of adhering to 'dying', 'death' and 'dead' to avoid confusion. For further reading look at Wentlandt et al. (2018) in the reference list.

References

Agar M et al. (2008). Preference for place of care and place of death in palliative care: are these different questions? *Palliative Medicine*, 22(7): 787–795.

Ariès P (1974). *Western Attitudes Towards Death: From the Middle Ages to the Present*. London: Marion Boyars.

Becker E (1973). *The Denial of Death*. New York: Free Press.

Corr CA (2016). Teaching about life and living in courses on death and dying. *Omega: Journal of Death and Dying*, 73(2): 174–187.

Cox K et al. (2013). Public attitudes to death and dying in the UK: a review of published literature. *BMJ Supportive & Palliative Care*, 3(1): 37.

Jull G (2017). Biopsychosocial model of disease: 40 years on. Which way is the pendulum swinging? *British Journal of Sports Medicine*, 51(16): 1187.

Kelemen A and Groninger H (2018). When we document end-of-life care, words still matter. *Journal of Pain and Symptom Management*, 57(1): e14.

Khoo Siew B (2005). The last hours and days of life: a biopsychosocial–spiritual model of care. *Asia Pacific Family Medicine*, 4: 1–3.

Kübler-Ross E (1970). *On Death and Dying*. New York: Collier Books/Macmillan Publishing Co.

Kusnanto H, Agustian D and Hilmanto D (2018). Biopsychosocial model of illnesses in primary care: a hermeneutic literature review. *Journal of Family Medicine and Primary Care*, 7(3): 497–500.

Llewellyn R et al. (2016). Cracking open death: death conversations in primary care. *Journal of Primary Health Care*, 8(4): 303–311.

Lutz D (2011). The dead still among us: Victorian secular relics, hair jewelry, and death culture. *Victorian Literature and Culture*, 39(1): 127–142.

McManus R (2012). *Death in a Global Age*. Basingstoke: Palgrave Macmillan.

Nebel Pederson S and Emmers-Sommer TM (2012). 'I'm not trying to be cured, so there's not much he can do for me': hospice patients' constructions of hospice's holistic care approach in a biomedical culture. *Death Studies*, 36(5): 419–446.

O'Meara P, Furness S and Gleeson R (2017). Educating paramedics for the future: a holistic approach. *Journal of Health and Human Services Administration*, 40(2): 219–251.

Pettifer A and Bronnert R (2013). End of life care in the community: the role of ambulance clinicians. *Journal of Paramedic Practice*, 5(7): 394–399.

Sayer D (2010). Who's afraid of the dead? Archaeology, modernity and the death taboo. *World Archaeology*, 42(3): 481–491.

SunLife (2018). *Cost of Dying Report 2018: A Complete View of Funeral Costs over Time*. Available at: https://www.sunlife.co.uk/siteassets/documents/cost-of-dying/cost-of-dying-report-2018.pdf.

Swetenham K, Grantham H and Glaetzer K (2014). Breaking down the silos: collaboration delivering an efficient and effective response to palliative care emergencies. *Progress in Palliative Care*, 22(4): 212–218.

Thulesius HO et al. (2013). De-tabooing dying control – A grounded theory study. *BMC Palliative Care*, 12(1): 13–20.

Wade DT and Halligan PW (2017). The biopsychosocial model of illness: a model whose time has come. *Clinical Rehabilitation*, 31(8): 995.

Walter T and Walter JA (1994). *The Revival of Death*. Hove: Psychology Press.

Walter T (2017a). Bodies and ceremonies: is the UK funeral industry still fit for purpose? *Mortality*, 22(3): 194–208.

Walter T (2017b). *What Death Means Now: Thinking Critically about Dying and Grieving*. Bristol: Policy Press.

Wentlandt K et al. (2018). Language used by health care professionals to describe dying at an acute care hospital. *Journal of Pain and Symptom Management*, 56(3): 337–343.

Yurevich A (2018). Attitudes to death as a scientific problem. *Herald of the Russian Academy of Sciences*, 88(1): 75–80.

Zimmermann C and Rodin G (2004). The denial of death thesis: sociological critique and implications for palliative care. *Palliative Medicine*, 18(2), 121–128.

Chapter 2

Defining Palliative Care
Tania Blackmore

Introduction

The terms we use to describe care of dying patients and those with incurable conditions are numerous. These terms include 'care of the dying', 'terminal care', 'hospice care', 'supportive care', 'end of life care' and 'palliative care'. The range and diversity of the terms used indicate the ever-changing societal attitudes towards palliative and end of life care, with 'softer' terms such as 'supportive care' greatly contrasting with terms such as 'care of the dying', while also showing its historical development as a health specialty (Gysels et al., 2013). Palliative care is usually considered to be the care of patients with an underlying life-limiting disease that cannot be cured, and end of life care is the care of patients in the last weeks, days and hours of life, so end of life care is considered to be the end of the disease trajectory of palliative care. Palliative care in the UK has developed rapidly over the last two decades and as such there are a range of tools and policies that concentrate on how the specialty is delivered across health sectors (Getty, 2018).

In order for the paramedic to understand the context of how palliative and end of life care is delivered, this chapter will look at the following essential international definitions, UK policies and care frameworks:

- The World Health Organization definition of palliative care
- The International Association for Hospice and Palliative Care definition of palliative care
- The foundation of the hospice movement in the UK
- The demise of the Liverpool Care Pathway
- One Chance to Get it Right document
- End of Life Care Strategy
- Gold Standards Framework
- Ambitions for Palliative and End of Life Care framework
- Recommended Summary Plan for Emergency Care and Treatment (ReSPECT)

- My Decisions

- The National Institute for Health and Care Excellence guidelines

- Advance care planning

- Paramedic practice and palliative care specifics.

Defining Palliative and End of Life Care

World Health Organization Definition and Principles of Palliative Care

The World Health Organization (WHO) suggests that palliative care incorporates the physical, psychosocial and spiritual problems of patients with life-limiting diseases and their loved ones, which cannot be achieved by one healthcare sector but needs the cooperation of a multi-disciplinary team (Borasio, 2011).

When explaining the extent of what palliative care encompasses, the WHO definition is usually given. Palliative care:

- provides relief from pain and other distressing symptoms

- affirms life and regards dying as a normal process

- intends neither to hasten nor postpone death

- integrates the psychological and spiritual aspects of patient care

- offers a support system to help patients live as actively as possible until death

- offers a support system to help the family cope during the patient's illness and in their own bereavement

- uses a team approach to address the needs of patients and their families, including bereavement counselling, if indicated

- will enhance quality of life, and may also positively influence the course of illness

- is applicable early in the course of illness, in conjunction with other therapies that are intended to prolong life, such as chemotherapy or radiation therapy, and includes those investigations needed to better understand and manage distressing clinical complications.

(World Health Organization, 2019)

The International Association for Hospice and Palliative Care Definition of Palliative Care

The International Association for Hospice and Palliative Care's recent definition of palliative care adapts the WHO definition and provides a more holistic approach to what palliative care entails.

Palliative care:

- includes, prevention, early identification, comprehensive assessment and management of physical issues, including pain and other distressing symptoms, psychological distress, spiritual distress and social needs. Whenever possible, these interventions must be evidence based

- provides support to help patients live as fully as possible until death by facilitating effective communication, helping them and their families determine goals of care

- is applicable throughout the course of an illness, according to the patient's needs

- is provided in conjunction with disease-modifying therapies whenever needed

- may positively influence the course of illness

- intends neither to hasten nor postpone death, affirms life, and recognises dying as a natural process

- provides support to the family and the caregivers during the patient's illness, and in their own bereavement

- is delivered recognising and respecting the cultural values and beliefs of the patient and the family

- is applicable throughout all healthcare settings (place of residence and institutions) and in all levels (primary to tertiary)

- can be provided by professionals with basic palliative care training

- requires specialist palliative care with a multiprofessional team for referral of complex cases.

(IAHPC, 2018)

The Foundation of the Hospice Movement

The founder of the hospice movement was Dame Cicely Saunders (Figure 2.1). She has been accredited with setting the standards of care and the philosophy that underpins palliative and end of life care not only in the UK but internationally. Cicely trained as a nurse at St Thomas's Hospital in the 1940s, but after a back injury she re-trained as a medical social worker, qualifying in 1947, and then studied as a doctor at St Thomas's, qualifying in 1957. It was in 1948 that she met Polish patient David Tasma at the Archway Hospital in London, and it was while caring for David, who was dying, that Cicely realised there was so much more that could be done for patients with a life-limiting prognosis. David and Cicely discussed the possibility of a home for dying patients, and in his will David left Cicely £500, a considerable sum at that time. David left the money with the comment 'I'll be a window in your home'. Cicely Saunders founded St Christopher's Hospice in 1967 in South West London, which was the first modern hospice. There is a window there dedicated to the memory of David Tasma.

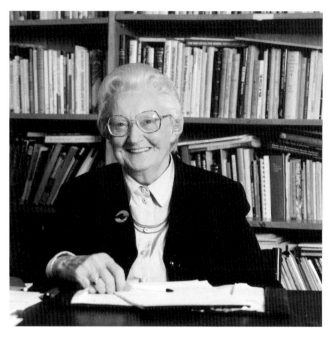

Figure 2.1 Dame Cicely Saunders, the founder of the hospice movement
Source: Reproduced with the kind permission of St Christopher's Hospice

Cicely Saunders promoted the idea that not achieving a cure for patients should not be seen as a failure in medicine. Healthcare should incorporate compassionate care, good symptom control, and respect and dignity for palliative and end of life patients as indicators of successful treatment. Her quote about the care of palliative and end of life patients is still today seen as the mission statement that guides all clinicians in palliative and end of life care:

> You matter because you are you, and you matter to the end of your life. We will do all we can not only to help you die peacefully, but also to live until you die.

> (Dame Cicely Saunders, nurse, physician,
> writer and founder of the hospice movement, 1918–2005)

It is important to note that the UK is still seen internationally to be at the forefront of palliative and end of life care due to the pioneering work of Cicely Saunders. In the *Quality of Death Index 2015*, a report by the Economist Intelligence Unit, the UK was ranked highest in quality of care of the dying and this was attributed to the National Health Service and the strong hospice movement founded by Cicely Saunders. The report also highlighted that even though the UK was rated the highest in the death index, there is evidence that the UK still does not adequately meet the needs of patients requiring palliative care (The Economist Intelligence Unit, 2015).

UK Policies and Frameworks in Palliative and End of Life Care

The Liverpool Care Pathway

The Liverpool Care Pathway (LCP) was a framework of care aimed at achieving good quality care for patients at the end of life. It was hoped that it would achieve hospice-like care within acute hospitals (Twigger and Yardley, 2017). Although the LCP was primarily formulated to be used in the acute sector, it was also used in community and hospice settings. It was introduced in the late 1990s and was in use until July 2014 when it was phased out in response to a growing anxiety from patients' families, health professionals and the media about its use, so much so that an independent review was undertaken (Twigger and Yardley, 2017). It is important to understand why the LCP failed in the context of current palliative and end of life policies so that the same mistakes are not made in current and future practice. The LCP is an example of where a framework went rogue and was not in the best interest of patient care.

The independent review of 2013, entitled 'More Care, Less Pathway' (DoH, 2013), chaired by Baroness Julia Neuberger, concluded that the LCP should be replaced by individualised patient plans for dying patients.

The independent review comments:

> Based on the evidence examined by the Review, much of which came from clinicians, the Review panel has concluded that the LCP is not being applied properly in all cases. Generic protocols, as the LCP has come to be seen, intended to be applicable for all patients in the last hours or days of their lives, in any setting, are the wrong approach. The Review panel strongly recommends the development of a series of guides and alerts that reflect the common principles of good palliative care, linking directly to the GMC's Guidance, and that of the NMC when it is developed. Implementation of this should be the personal responsibility of clinicians. The Review panel envisages that, in addition to the core driving palliative care philosophy that will be common to all guidance, there would be elements of technical guidance specific to certain disease groups, such as solid cancers, haematological cancers and other blood diseases, organ failure and cardio-respiratory diseases, neurological conditions, respiratory conditions, and for patients with dementia. An important requirement for these guidelines is that they be designed to be readily adapted for local use to meet the needs of individuals.
>
> (DoH, 2013)

It can be said that the LCP was a classic example of the old saying that 'one size does not fit all' and that if we are to achieve the best care for palliative and end of life patients that we need to view our patients as individuals with unique needs.

The Liverpool Care Pathway is often cited in research as an example of the dangers of implementing a treatment framework or pathway without basing an intervention on hard clinical evidence, and there was very little research that examined the benefits of its use in the care of the dying (Seymour and Clark, 2018; Twigger and Yardley, 2017).

One Chance to Get It Right Document

This document was published in June 2014 by the Leadership Alliance for the Care of Dying People (LACDP), a coalition of 21 national organisations that was set up to improve the care of the dying patient following the independent review of the Liverpool Care Pathway. The document set up priorities of care that should be followed by clinicians if a person was expected to die within the next few days or hours.

Priorities for Care of the Dying Person

1. The possibility (that a person may die within the next few days or hours) is recognised and communicated clearly, decisions made, and actions taken in accordance with the person's needs and wishes, and these are regularly reviewed, and decisions revised accordingly.

2. Sensitive communication takes place between staff and the dying person, and those identified as important to them.

3. The dying person, and those identified as important to them, are involved in decisions about treatment and care to the extent that the dying person wishes.

4. The needs of families and others identified as important to the dying person are actively explored, respected and met as far as possible.

5. An individual plan of care, which includes food and drink, symptom control and psychological, social and spiritual support, is agreed, coordinated and delivered with compassion.

All health and care staff who care for dying patients must ensure that they are aware of and follow up-to-date guidance and local best practice. They must recognise that the evidence on which this is based will continue to evolve, so a commitment to lifelong learning is fundamental.

One Chance to Get it Right

The guidance from the Leadership Alliance for the Care of Dying People document was less specific than the LCP and promoted multi-disciplinary working across health sectors and among healthcare professionals, as opposed to the rigid algorithms seen in the LCP. The priorities of care for the dying patient will be discussed in greater detail in Chapter 6 – Care of the Dying Patient.

End of Life Care Strategy

When discussing relevant policies, it is important to acknowledge the role of the UK's End of Life Care Strategy (EOLCS), which was commissioned by the government to come up with a plan to coordinate services for dying people, regardless of the disease or condition they are suffering from (Department of Health, 2008).

> ... [helping] all those with advanced, progressive, incurable illness to live as well as possible until they die. It enables the supportive and palliative care needs of both patient and family to be identified and met throughout the last phase of life and into bereavement. It includes management of pain and other symptoms and provision of psychological, social, spiritual and practical support.
>
> (DoH, 2008: 47)

The EOLCS proposed a six-step approach to ensure good quality care at end of life:

Step 1 – Discussions as the end of life approaches.

Step 2 – Assessment, care planning and review.

Step 3 – Coordination of care for individual patients.

Step 4 – Delivery of high-quality services in different settings.

Step 5 – Care in the last days of life.

Step 6 – Care after death.

(DoH, 2008: 48)

The EOLCS promoted equality of care at end of life not only for all causes of death but for all health sectors, and outlined the entitlements of dying patients and their loved ones as follows:

- Patients have their needs assessed by a professional or professionals with appropriate expertise.
- Patients have a care plan that records their preferences and the choices they would like to make.
- The care plan should be reviewed as the patient's condition changes.
- Patients should be involved in decisions about treatments prescribed for them, including the option to say 'no' to treatments they do not wish to have prescribed.
- Patients and their loved ones should know that systems are in place to ensure that information about patients' needs and preferences can be accessed by all relevant health and social care staff with their permission.

(DoH, 2008: 56)

A national programme was launched to underpin the EOLCS and the government invested nearly £300 million establishing this programme, which stated that primary care trusts (PCTs) should have a defined plan on how they would achieve the six steps (Learner, 2011). The overriding opinion seems to be that the EOLCS did raise the profile of care of the dying in the public and clinician's awareness, but it is hard to assess whether this influenced or improved the care of the dying. A criticism of the EOLCS was its use of tools that included the LCP and the Gold Standards Framework, which have little evidence or evaluation of the benefits of their use (Ingleton et al., 2009). It has been suggested that EOLCS improved satisfaction of bereaved relatives of patients that died at home, but the implementation of the strategy in hospitals was slower, which resulted in bereaved relatives of patients who were cared for in the hospital setting reporting less satisfaction, and as the hospital is the most common place to die, there is still work to be done regarding a national pathway that is effective across all health sectors (Triggle, 2012).

Gold Standards Framework

The Gold Standards Framework (GSF) is widely used in primary care settings in the UK. It was developed in 2000, initially by GP Keri Thomas, who had a special interest in palliative and end of life care and started a project that was considered on review to have been a great success for patient care so was rolled out nationally (Shaw et al., 2010). It is primarily a screening tool for patients who have a life-limiting illness and is initiated by the GP looking at all the patients on their caseload and asking the question 'would you be surprised if this patient died in the next year?'. If the answer is 'no', then the GSF should be implemented for that patient (O'Callaghan et al., 2014). The GSF dictates that those patients who are categorised as 'gold patients' should be prioritised when seeking help and should be offered extra support from primary care. This extra support is sometimes referral by the GP to the community palliative care team at the local hospice for emotional or symptom control support. The gold patient and potential gold patients are discussed in a monthly multidisciplinary team meeting held at the GP surgery and attended by representatives of the community social work team, the district nurse team, the GP medical team and a clinical nurse specialist from the hospice to ensure that the patient has an effective coordinated care programme. The GSF should be a programme that incorporates the following:

1. Identifies patients in the last years of life.
2. Assesses their needs, symptoms and preferences.
3. Enables patients to plan and choose where they want to live and die.

(Shaw et al., 2010)

A review of the GSF has concluded that the GSF has been effective in improving end of life care, but there is still room for improvement and more government investment is needed to accommodate the ageing UK population (Shaw et al., 2010).

The GSF promotes training of all staff that care for patients at the end of life, promoting the organisation of care through cooperation across different health sectors, and is a useful resource for any clinician wanting further information about end of life care. The GSF mission statement is as follows:

> Our aspiration is to deliver training and support that brings about individual and organisational transformation, enabling a 'gold standard' of care for all people nearing the end of life.

(The Gold Standards Framework, 2019)

Ambitions for Palliative and End of Life Care (2015)

This report was underpinned by the values outlined in the GSF and written by The National Palliative and End of Life Partnership, which consists of a group of national organisations that have experience and responsibility for the care of palliative and end of life patients. These organisations included the Association of Ambulance Chief Executives as well as the Royal College of Physicians, the Royal College of Nursing, Hospice UK and Macmillan Cancer Support.

The report identified six ambitions from the viewpoint of the dying patient.

1. Each person is seen as an individual.

2. Each person gets fair access to care.

3. Maximisation of comfort and wellbeing.

4. Care is coordinated.

5. All staff are prepared to care.

6. Each community is prepared to help.

(Adapted from National Partnership for Palliative and End of Life Care, 2015)

This report outlined a national framework that should be used to implement good quality palliative and end of life care across all health settings incorporating the recommendations of the past policies in palliative care such as the Leadership Alliance Report, the review of the LCP and the GSF (Wee, 2016). Reading this report is recommended as it provides excellent guidance and resources for the paramedic in the care of the dying patient, with an emphasis on the inequalities that exist for dying patients in their access to good quality care. It is one of the few policies that included the viewpoint of paramedic practice by involving the Association of Ambulance Chief Executives as part of the advisory panel.

ReSPECT

ReSPECT is a process that aims to formulate a personal plan for the future for individuals that have life-limiting conditions. The acronym stands for Recommended Summary Plan for Emergency Care and Treatment. It is a form that has been implemented in some areas of the UK as part of a formal research evaluation over three years that contains the following information about the patient:

1. Personal details.

2. Summary of relevant information.

3. Personal preferences.

4. Clinical recommendation for emergency care treatment.

5. Capacity of the patient at the time of completing the form.

6. Who was involved in completing the form.

7. Clinician's signature.

8. Emergency contacts.

9. Confirmation of validity.

(Resuscitation Council UK, 2020)

Plans such as ReSPECT are considered to be useful tools for people with life-limiting conditions, conditions that are predisposed to sudden cardiac arrest, or a long-term condition that causes a sudden deterioration (Pitcher et al., 2017). It is important to note the difference between an anticipatory or advance care plan (ACP) and an emergency care plan. An ACP usually records the patient's treatment and care wishes with an emphasis on end of life care and choices, whereas an emergency plan provides precise clinical recommendation in an emergency (Pitcher et al., 2017). Please see the section on ACP in this chapter and be aware that often ACP and emergency plans can be used alongside each other to achieve the best patient care at end of life. A combination of the patient's choices and clinical expertise in end of life care has been found to be the best way to achieve the best care for dying patients (Land et al., 2019). The partnership between patient and clinician is fundamental to the principles and guidelines in palliative and end of life care. As stated earlier ReSPECT has unfortunately not been implemented across the UK as yet, but it is hoped that the process will gradually become more widely adopted so as to avoid any potential gaps in coverage for paramedics and their patients. The ReSPECT website recommends the use of My Decisions (2020) for patients not in areas covered by the ReSPECT implementation. This website provides an advance care plan that can be completed online by the patient or a form that can be downloaded. This produces a document that when signed and witnessed is a legal document of the patient's wishes.

The National Institute for Health and Care Excellence guidelines

NICE provides guidelines on different aspects of palliative and end of life care, including administration of opioids at end of life and guidance for the end stages of specific cancers and long-term conditions. The most pertinent guidelines are cited and described below.

Caring for an Adult at the End of Life

The following are NICE guideline statements on 'Care of dying adults in the last days of life.

> **Statement 1**: Adults who have signs and symptoms that suggest they may be in the last days of life are monitored for further changes to help determine if they are nearing death, stabilising or recovering.

> **Statement 2:** Adults in the last days of life, and the people important to them, are given opportunities to discuss, develop and review an individualised care plan.

Statement 3: Adults in the last days of life who are likely to need symptom control are prescribed anticipatory medicines with individualised indications for use, dosage and route of administration.

Statement 4: Adults in the last days of life have their hydration status assessed daily and discuss the risks and benefits of hydration options.

(NICE, 2011)

These statements mirror the aims and priorities of other national end of life care policies by an emphasis on symptom control, communication, care planning and the discussion of nutrition at end of life. The chapters of this book also cover the topics outlined by the national policies.

In addition to the NICE guideline on 'End of life care for adults: quality standard', NICE provides two further guidelines on pain relief and end of life care in chronic conditions which provide evidence-based symptom control guidance which are useful to paramedic practice. These are specific National Institute for Health and Care Excellence guidelines that relate to end of life care and stipulate what should be addressed in the palliative and end of life patient, as follows:

Opioids for Pain Relief in Palliative Care

1. Starting strong opioids, titration and dose.

2. Managing common symptoms.

3. Oral morphine.

4. Transdermal patches or subcutaneous delivery.

5. Breakthrough pain.

End of Life Care for People with Life-Limiting Conditions

1. Agitation.

2. Pain.

3. Respiratory distress.

4. Seizure.

5. Unresolved distressing symptoms.

Preferred Place of Care and Advance Care Planning

A theme that runs through all end of life and palliative care policies is a need to plan and achieve patient preferences about where they want to be cared for and where they want to die: this is known predominantly as 'Preferred Place of Care' or 'Priorities of Care'. There is a clear discrepancy in the UK between a person's preferred place of death and where they actually die with statistics showing that 70% of people want to die at home but 50% of people still actually die in hospital (Arnold et al., 2015; McCaughan et al., 2019). Research indicates that the transition from palliative care to end of life care is hard to identify for generalist clinicians and as a consequence patients are not identified as in the end stages of life, and so their places of death are not being achieved (Gott et al., 2011). To achieve preferred place of care and death it is imperative that palliative patients have participated in advance care planning, so their wishes have been documented at a time that they are physically and emotionally capable of doing so, which protects the patient at a time in the future when, because of emotional and physical fragility, they can no longer express themselves. Advance Care Planning (ACP) is often confusing and hard to define because of the array of different terms and forms it may take in palliative care but the term encompasses advance decisions, preferred places of care and all plans made in advance of a patient's deterioration at end of life (Russell, 2018). Advance decisions, also known as advance directives or living wills, identify situations in which the patient would or would not want specified treatments. Please refer to Chapter 7 – Ethics for more detail on the difference between advance care planning and advance directives. Looking at the research on preferred place of care and advance care planning there are three prominent themes that emerge and need to be considered.

1. **The need for increased communication in palliative care.** Merryn Gott et al. (2011) outlined poor communication by clinicians to relatives and carers of dying palliative patients, even at the very end stage of the patient's life. Slatyer et al. (2013) suggested that lack of communication between the acute sector and the community sector led to avoidable admissions of palliative patients into hospital. No information was given by acute clinicians to palliative patients and their carers about their discharge and care needs, leading to palliative patients feeling disempowered and out of control (Slatyer et al., 2013). Research indicates that when palliative patients are admitted to the emergency department, the emergency clinicians have little information about these patients, which leads to a defensive and biomedical approach to their care, and which also generates multiple inappropriate investigations and tests (Grudzen et al., 2012).

2. **The need for advance care planning in palliative care.** Gott et al. (2013) indicated that in their sample of 183 palliative patients there was no evidence of individualised advance care planning, even though the End of Life Care Strategy (DoH, 2008) highlighted the need for advance care planning for palliative patients and the importance of multidisciplinary working and interprofessional information sharing. Hussain et al. (2013) emphasised that palliative patients who have an individual plan or pathway are less likely to be admitted to hospital than those who don't.

3. **The need for multidisciplinary working in palliative care.** Advance care planning enables increased communication across healthcare sectors. If a

palliative patient has their notes with them, these are available both in the hospital and in the community for all clinicians including paramedics to share (Blackmore, 2016). Community clinicians such as paramedics should be more aware of their roles in providing treatment for palliative and end of life patients in order to to enable certain patients to remain at home. This lessens the likelihood of admission increasing in the last week of the patient's life, which is currently the case (Robinson et al., 2018).

Paramedic Practice and Palliative Care Specifics

A recent study emphasises that unnecessary admissions of end of life patients to hospital is not only a UK but an international problem (Hoare et al., 2018). Paramedics reported positively about enabling patients to die at home but stated there were barriers to achieving this, such as arranging out of hours care for patients at end of life, scarce patient information available to paramedics and an ambulance service that had a treatment protocol based on emergency care not palliative care (Hoare et al., 2018). For more information about advance care plans and advance directives, please look at Chapter 6 – Care of the Dying Patient and Chapter 7 – Ethics.

What Is Already Known About the Topic?

1. Hospital admissions immediately prior to the end of life are considered negatively in many policy documents, with home assumed to be a better place to die.

2. Ambulance staff struggle with limited patient information and the need to make time-critical decisions when caring for end of life patients.

3. Little is known about why end of life patient ambulance transfers to hospital occur (Hoare et al., 2018). Paramedics need the training, information and support to be able to manage the distressing symptoms of patients at end of life, to uphold the wishes of dying patients and also have the confidence to deal successfully with the emotional needs of the family of the dying patients. The competencies needed by paramedics to achieve good care of dying patients can be summarised into four themes:

    a. **Multifocal assessment** – this may also be described as holistic assessment that incorporates the care of the family as well as the patient.

    b. **Family responses** – responding to the emotional needs of the loved ones and family members who are present.

    c. **Conflicts** – adhering to 'do not resuscitate' orders or not, and arbitrating in family disputes.

    d. **Management of the dying process** – symptom control and clinical decision making in a holistic manner (Waldrop et al., 2015).

It is hoped that after reading this book, engaging in further reading and looking at the provided case studies, you will gain more confidence as a paramedic in dealing with these themes.

> ### *Pause for thought*
>
> Consider where you would prefer to be cared for at end of life?
>
> Explain the following:
>
> 1. Why you have chosen this preference?
> 2. Would you be influenced by your family, especially if they did not want you to die in your preferred place?
> 3. What factors might impact your family in concern to where you die?
>
> This is difficult to think about but please remember it's as hard for you to consider as your patient; when a patient receives a palliative prognosis, their hopes and aspirations don't disappear with their prognosis.

References

Arnold E, Finucane AM and Oxenham D (2015). Preferred place of death for patients referred to a specialist palliative care service. *BMJ Supportive and Palliative Care*, 5(3): 294.

Blackmore TA (2016). What are the opinions of acute clinicians of patient held records for palliative patients? *European Journal of Palliative Care*, 23(3): 118–123.

Borasio GD (2011). Translating the World Health Organization definition of palliative care into scientific practice. *Palliative and Supportive Care*, 9(1): 1–2.

Department of Health (2008). *End of Life Care Strategy: Promoting High Quality Care for All Adults at End of Life*. London: HMSO.

Department of Health (2013). *More Care, Less Pathway: A Review of the Liverpool Care Pathway*. 1st ed. [eBook], 6–63. Available at: https://www.gov.uk/government/uploads/system/uploads/attachment_data/file/212450/Liverpool_Care_Pathway.pdf.

Economist Intelligence Unit (2015). *The Quality of Death Index*. Available at: https://eiuperspectives.economist.com/sites/default/files/2015%20EIU%20Quality%20of%20Death%20Index%20Oct%2029%20FINAL.pdf.

Getty J (2018). Principles of Palliative Care. *InnovAiT*, 11(12): 676–679.

Gold Standards Framework (2019). *The A programme for community palliative care*. Available at: www.goldstandardsframework.org.uk/.

Gott M et al. (2011). Transitions to palliative care in acute hospitals in England: qualitative study. *BMJ Supportive and Palliative Care*, 1(1): 42.

Gott M et al. (2013). Transitions to palliative care for older people in acute hospitals: a mixed-methods study. *Health Services and Delivery Research*, 1(11).

Grudzen CR et al. (2012). Does palliative care have a future in the emergency department? Discussions with attending emergency physicians. *Journal of Pain and Symptom Management*, 43(1): 1–9.

Gysels M et al. (2013). Diversity in defining end of life care: an obstacle or the way forward? *PLoS ONE*, 8(7): e68002.

Hoare S et al. (2018). Ambulance staff and end-of-life hospital admissions: a qualitative interview study. *Palliative Medicine*, 32(9): 1465–1473.

Hussain JA, Mooney A and Russon L (2013). Comparison of survival analysis and palliative care involvement in patients aged over 70 years choosing conservative management or renal replacement therapy in advanced chronic kidney disease. *Palliative Medicine*, 27(9): 829.

IAHPC (2018). Global Consensus based palliative care definition. Houston, TX: The International Association for Hospice and Palliative Care. Available at: https://hospicecare.com/what-we-do/projects/consensus-based-definition-of-palliative-care/definition/.

Ingleton C, Gott M and Kirk S (2009). Editorial: The beginning of the end (of life care strategy). *Journal of Clinical Nursing*, 18(7): 935–937.

Land V et al. (2019). Addressing possible problems with patients' expectations, plans and decisions for the future: one strategy used by experienced clinicians in advance care planning conversations. *Patient Education and Counseling*, 102(4): 670.

Leadership Alliance for the Care of Dying People (2014). *One chance to get it right: improving people's experience of care in the last few days and hours of life*. Available at: https://assets.publishing.service.gov.uk/government/uploads/system/uploads/attachment_data/file/323188/One_chance_to_get_it_right.pdf.

Learner S (2011). A better death: three years after its launch, Sue Learner asks if the end of life care strategy has improved services. *Nursing Standard*, 25(35): 20.

McCaughan D et al. (2019). Perspectives of bereaved relatives of patients with haematological malignancies concerning preferred place of care and death: a qualitative study. *Palliative Medicine*, 33(5): 518–530.

My Decisions (2020). *My Decisions*. Available at: https://mydecisions.org.uk/.

National Institute for Health and Care Excellence (2011). *End of life care for adults: quality standard [QS13]*. Available at: https://www.nice.org.uk/guidance/qs13.

National Partnership for Palliative and End of Life Care (2015). *Ambitions for palliative and end of life care: a national framework for local action: 2015–2020*. Available at: http://endoflifecareambitions.org.uk/.

O'Callaghan A et al. (2014). Can we predict which hospitalised patients are in their last year of life? A prospective cross-sectional study of the Gold Standards Framework Prognostic Indicator Guidance as a screening tool in the acute hospital setting. *Palliative Medicine*, 28(8): 1046–1052.

Pitcher D et al. (2017). Emergency care and resuscitation plans. *BMJ*, 356: j876.

Resuscitation Council UK (2020). *ReSPECT*. Available at: https://www.resus.org.uk/respect/.

Robinson J et al. (2018). Circumstances of hospital admissions in palliative care: a cross-sectional survey of patients admitted to hospital with palliative care needs. *Palliative Medicine*, 32(5): 1030–1036.

Seymour J and Clark D (2018). The Liverpool Care Pathway for the Dying Patient: a critical analysis of its rise, demise and legacy in England. *Wellcome Open Research*, 3: 15–15.

Shaw K et al. (2010). Review: Improving end-of-life care: a critical review of the Gold Standards Framework in primary care. *Palliative Medicine*, 24(3): 317–329.

Slatyer S et al. (2013). Early re-presentation to hospital after discharge from an acute medical unit: perspectives of older patients, their family caregivers and health professionals. *Journal of Clinical Nursing*, 22(3–4): 445–455.

Triggle N (2012). End of life care strategy to focus on standards in hospital. *Nursing Older People*, 24(10): 6–7.

Twigger S and Yardley SJ (2017). Hospital doctors' understanding of use and withdrawal of the Liverpool Care Pathway: a qualitative study of practice-based experiences during times of change. *Palliative Medicine*, 31(9): 833–841.

Waldrop DP et al. (2015). 'We are strangers walking into their life-changing event': how prehospital providers manage emergency calls at the end of life. *Journal of Pain and Symptom Management*, 50(3): 328–334.

Wee B (2016). Ambitions for palliative and end-of-life care. *Clinical Medicine (London, England)*, 16(3): 213–214.

World Health Organization (2019). *Who Definition of Palliative Care*. Available at: https://www.who .int/cancer/palliative/definition/en/.

Chapter 3

Palliative Care Emergencies

Fiona Kiely

Introduction

While the majority of paramedics have had professional experience of palliative emergency situations, there is a paucity of supporting guidelines or educational programmes to guide or support these uniquely placed healthcare professionals who are integral to the community–hospital interface and, indeed, the community provision of palliative care (Donnelly et al., 2015; Wiese et al., 2008; Wiese et al., 2013). Given that 3–10% of all pre-hospital emergencies qualify as palliative emergencies, it represents a significant area of complex healthcare provision in need of support (Wiese et al., 2013). The JRCALC guidelines (2019) offer guidance on specific palliative emergencies including metastatic spinal cord compression, superior vena cava compression and neutropenic sepsis so do refer to this along with local trust guidance. Paramedics should be aware of their own scope of practice when managing palliative emergencies and also abide their local NHS trust guidance.

Currow and Clark (2006) also provide a useful clinical decision-making framework for guiding good palliative practice for healthcare professionals: the WHY framework. It is relevant to the paramedic assessing a patient experiencing a palliative emergency, as it provides fundamental questions to inform good practice.

Underpinning this framework is the importance of asking the question 'Why?' when assessing a change in the clinical condition of a patient and deciding on emergency (or any) management plans. Knowing the anticipated and natural course of the illness is key to recognising an unexpected change that may represent a palliative emergency. All unexpected changes need to be carefully assessed. It is necessary to consider whether this new presentation is:

- An expected manifestation of the disease
- An unexpected manifestation of the disease
- An exacerbation of an intercurrent problem
- A new intercurrent problem.

Essentially, the crucial question to ask is:

> ### WHY is this person unwell today?
>
> Is it because of overall anticipated progression of maximally treated disease [an expected deterioration given the natural history and prognosis of the disease]?
>
> OR
>
> Is it because of the effects of an acute problem that can reasonably be reversed [an unexpected deterioration given the natural history and prognosis of the disease]? (Currow and Clark, 2006)

An understanding of the natural history and prognosis of the disease, albeit of a life-limiting nature, may need recalibration in view of the effects of novel therapeutics in advanced illness coupled with the earlier integration of palliative care in serious illness which is no longer synonymous with care just at the very end of life (Parikh et al., 2013; Temel et al., 2010). Patients with palliative care needs are at risk of developing reversible life-altering or life-limiting problems which, if addressed, may maintain an acceptable quality of life as determined by the patient or extend survival. The best symptom control remains, where possible, to treat the underlying cause of the symptom (Currow and Clark, 2006).

Conversely, just because we can do something about the problem does not necessarily mean we should. In palliative care situations, the response to such emergency situations is informed by the patient's clinical context, rather than just the event itself.

Decisions around management and what action to take should incorporate consideration of the:

- Natural history and prognosis of the disease
- Performance status and general condition of the patient
- Patient and family wishes, including advance care plans or directives
- Burden versus benefit of treatment: how likely is it to be reversed
- Symptom burden of the illness.

(Fowell and Stuart, 2011; Watson, 2009)

Merging the above considerations will begin to provide a framework within which to approach palliative emergencies. While there are a myriad of urgencies and emergencies in palliative care contexts, the focus in this chapter is on four of the more common, but potentially reversible, emergencies requiring urgent and prompt diagnosis and management. The chapter also deals with catastrophic events in terminal patients and how to manage these events when they arise. The palliative care emergencies discussed in this chapter are as follows:

- Superior vena cava syndrome
- Malignant hypercalcaemia
- Metastatic spinal cord compression
- Neutropenic sepsis
- Catastrophic events in terminal patients.

Superior Vena Cava Syndrome

Background

Superior vena cava syndrome (SVCS) is a clinical condition resulting from partial or complete obstruction of blood flow through the superior vena cava (SVC), the blood vessel responsible for carrying one third of the total venous return to the heart (Wilson et al., 2007). This obstruction may be caused by compression, invasion, thrombosis or fibrosis of this thin-walled vessel (Halfdanarson et al., 2017). It is a potential complication of cancer, with malignancies accounting for most cases. The most common malignant causes are non-small cell lung cancer (approximately 50% of patients), small cell lung cancers (25% of patients), followed by lymphoma and metastatic lesions. It is the presenting feature of a previously unknown tumour in 60% of cases. The syndrome is increasingly seen as a complication of benign aetiology, partly reflecting increased use of intravascular devices such as catheters, pacemakers, implantable cardioverter-defibrillators and cardiac resynchronisation therapy (Lewis et al., 2011). Symptoms develop over a two-week period in a third of patients, and over longer periods of time in the remaining cases. The speed of onset and severity of symptoms dictates the urgency of intervention. SVCS causes significant patient distress, usually heralds a serious underlying condition, and warrants expedient management as it may be life threatening in certain instances (Straka et al., 2016).

Impact

Prognosis typically depends on the underlying cause, with poor outcome for malignant conditions (Straka et al., 2016). In patients with treatment-responsive malignancies, the occurrence of SVCS does not necessarily adversely affect their overall survival (Sculier et al., 1986). However, in patients whose cancer is resistant to chemotherapy or radiotherapy, the development of SVCS confers a poor prognosis and median survival less than six months (Rowell and Gleeson, 2002).

SVCS may be life-threatening in rare cases and in such instances, it requires urgent treatment. The presence of laryngeal or cerebral oedema in particular require prompt management and rapid treatment of the underlying cause of SVCS. If left untreated, consequences include death or long-term morbidity impairing function and quality of life. SVCS relapse rates are low following radiotherapy, chemotherapy or stenting (Straka et al., 2016). These treatments are effective for symptom control and can control symptoms within hours to weeks depending on the chosen modality.

The treatments for SVCS are generally well tolerated and successful but as with all treatments, are not without potential morbidity. An uncommon but serious complication of stent placement in long-term survivors is stent migration. Stents may also require the patient to be on anti-thrombotic therapy for a period of time (Schifferdecker et al., 2005). The usual potential side effects of radiotherapy and chemotherapy apply.

Pathophysiology and Clinical Aspects

The SVC is the blood vessel that carries blood from the head, arms and upper torso to the heart. It is located in the central compartment of the thoracic cavity, known as the mediastinum and is surrounded by structures including the trachea, right bronchus, aorta, pulmonary artery and lymph nodes. Compression of the SVC can be caused by tumours or masses located within the mediastinum, generally to the right of the midline (Figure 3.1). As mentioned already, this type of external compression is not the only cause of SVCS – thrombosis, fibrosis and infiltration of the vessel are other causes.

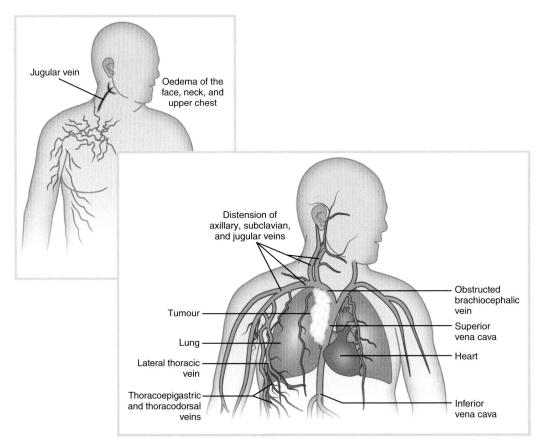

Figure 3.1 Superior vena cava syndrome

When the SVC is blocked, venous pressure rises in the upper body, resulting in swelling of the head, neck and arms, often with cyanosis, facial redness and distended subcutaneous vessels. This swelling may compromise the larynx or pharynx causing cough, hoarseness, dyspnoea, stridor and dysphagia. Swelling affecting the brain may lead to headache, confusion, seizures and coma (Wilson et al., 2007) The extent and rapidity of narrowing of the vessel dictates the nature and severity of how the patient presents (Lewis et al., 2011). When obstruction occurs abruptly it can be florid in its presentation and constitute a medical emergency due to laryngeal or cerebral swelling. However, symptoms of SVCS more typically present insidiously over a period of days or weeks.

Slowly progressive obstruction allows time for blood to find and create alternative ways of reaching the heart – a 'collateral' circulation system is developed to accommodate the blood flow of the superior vena cava. This requires a period of a few weeks to evolve and it may be seen as abnormal distension and dilation of neck and upper torso vessels (Figure 3.1). Due to the reduced venous return to the heart in SVCS, haemodynamic instability may ensue (Wilson et al., 2007).

How Do I Recognise It?

SVCS may have an insidious onset and so can be difficult to recognise initially. Consideration should be given to the WHY framework, risk factors for SVCS, in combination with a thorough history and relevant examination (Currow and Clark, 2006).

> **Step 1.** Identify the presence of risk factors:
>
> - commonly associated malignancies shown in Table 3.1 (but remember 60% of cases present as new cancer)
>
> - previous intravascular procedures.
>
> **Step 2.** Targeted history and examination.

Table 3.1 Malignancies associated with developing SVCS

Tumour Type	Proportion	Suggestive Clinical Features
Non-small cell lung cancer	50%	History of smoking, age often >50 years
Small cell lung cancer	22%	History of smoking, age often >50 years
Lymphoma	12%	Enlarged nodes, age often <65 years
Metastatic cancer	9%	Often occurs in breast cancer

(Based on Currow and Clark, 2006)

As a paramedic attending an emergency call, a clinical diagnosis of SVCS will be made on the basis of signs and symptoms. The presentation most commonly evolves over a period of days to weeks and may be clinically striking. The clinical features of SVCS are considered in Table 3.2.

Table 3.2 Signs and symptoms of SVCS

Sign or Symptom	Frequency %	Implication
Facial swelling	82	Increased venous pressure
Arm swelling	46	Increased venous pressure
Distended neck veins	63	Increased venous pressure
Distended chest veins	53	Increased venous pressure
Facial plethora	20	Increased venous pressure
Visual symptoms	2	Increased venous pressure
Dyspnoea	54	Laryngeal compromise, tumour
Cough	54	Laryngeal compromise
Hoarseness	17	Laryngeal compromise
Stridor	4	Laryngeal compromise
Collapse	10	Cerebral oedema, haemodynamic compromise
Headaches, dizziness, confusion	18	Cerebral oedema, haemodynamic compromise
Obtundation (altered level of consciousness)	2	Cerebral oedema

(Based on Currow and Clark, 2006)

With slow onset SVCS, the patient may complain of upper body or face swelling (which may be worse in the morning), headache or 'fullness' on bending or lying down, and increasing dyspnoea. In acute onset SVCS, complaints of dizziness and sudden onset dyspnoea are common (Currow and Clark, 2006).

Physical examination may be notable for dilated veins on neck, forehead, anterior chest wall. The patient's eyes may appear bloodshot in association with facial swelling (Figure 3.2 and Figure 3.3).

Assessment may reveal tachypnoea, swelling of arms, face or neck and peripheral cyanosis. Pemberton's sign may be present if an obstruction of the inlet to the thorax is causing SVCS. This sign is elicited by asking the patient to raise both arms above their head. Facial congestion develops on arm raising and disappears again on lowering the arms.

Airway patency should be assessed as laryngeal oedema may cause life-threatening respiratory compromise. Cerebral function also requires assessment because cerebral oedema may manifest in acute onset SVCS.

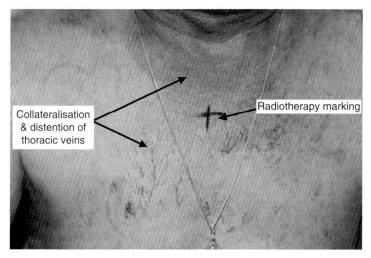

Figure 3.2 Venous distension in SVCS

Source: Author's image of patient. Reproduced with the patient's full consent

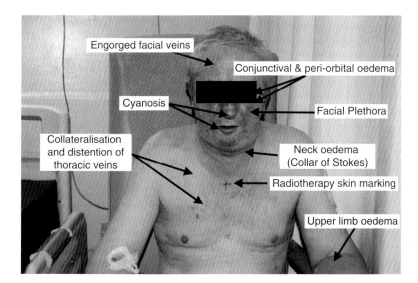

Figure 3.3 Clinical signs in SVCS

Source: Author's image of patient. Reproduced with the patient's full consent

Management

When SVCS is clinically suspected, decisions need to be made regarding how best to manage the palliative emergency (Table 3.3).

When treatment is appropriate and desired:

1. If any of the following time-critical features present:

   a. major airway, breathing, circulation (ABC) problems

   b. stridor or severe respiratory distress

      c. altered consciousness

           i. start correcting ABC problems

          ii. undertake a time-critical transfer to nearest emergency department. Provide patient management en route

        iii. provide an alert/information call.

2. In the absence of the above time-critical features, elevate the patient's head or sit the patient upright to decrease hydrostatic pressure. This may provide symptomatic relief.

3. Administer supplemental oxygen if patient has low O_2 saturations.

4. Transfer to the nearest emergency department or to a specialist unit if advised by a specialist team.

Table 3.3 Relevant considerations for treatment of SVCS

Context and Considerations	Potential Actions and Outcomes
Natural history and prognosis of disease prior to emergency	<ul><li>If prognosis measured in hours to days prior to onset of this problem, then the focus is on symptom control.</li><li>For example, opioids will be necessary for management of dyspnoea and headache, supplemental oxygen may be required if the patient is breathless and hypoxaemic, benzodiazepines may be necessary for anxiety and seizure management. Acute airway compromise may require use of crisis medications for this terminal event.</li><li>While it may be preferable for symptom control of the dying patient in the last hours/days of life to continue at home, it is important to understand that sometimes the severity of symptoms or care needs are beyond what can reasonably be managed at home and specialist support is necessary. This may require a transfer to an acute hospital setting or hospice, or arrangement of specialist nursing input in the home, for example.</li><li>Patients with prognoses of weeks, months or years prior to onset of this problem should, in addition to symptom control, be investigated and treated for suspected SVCS.</li><li>Because the symptoms of SVCS can be distressing and are likely to respond to treatment, pursuing the diagnosis should be seriously considered even for those with limited overall prognosis of weeks.</li></ul>

Context and Considerations	Potential Actions and Outcomes
Performance status and general condition of patient	• Consider how treatment of SVCS may preserve or improve the performance status of the patient. • Does the general condition of the patient permit transfer to a hospital?
Patient and family wishes	• Do patient and family desire the anticipated treatment and have they received sufficient information to make an informed decision (refer to 'Impact of SVCS' above)? • Check the patient's capacity for decision making. • Check if an Advance Care Directive specifically addresses this circumstance.
Burden versus benefit treatment	• Burden of treatment – generally well tolerated. Major complications with stenting are rare and include stent migration, pulmonary emboli, vessel rupture and pericardial tamponade. • Potential benefits include resolution of burdensome SVCS symptoms (see Table 3.2) and better survival benefit conferred when treated rather than untreated. • Stenting is very successful technically and relieves symptoms in hours to days. • In the cases where chemotherapy or radiotherapy is the treatment choice for SVCS, a response can be expected in 50–70% of patients within 2–3 weeks. When radiotherapy is palliative, the course of treatment is typically over 1–3 weeks, with daily fractionation.
Will treatment improve quality of life?	• What would treatment actually change for the patient? How much value does the patient place on that change? This is very individual.

In-Hospital Treatment

In the case of malignant causes of SVCS, management involves both treatment of the cancer in addition to relief of symptoms of obstruction. The strategy adopted is guided by the severity of symptoms, the nature of the malignancy, as well as the anticipated response to treatment. Steroids and diuretics are commonly used to reduce oedema and venous pressure, but the evidence base for these approaches is weak. Traditionally, superior vena cava syndrome has been managed with radiotherapy and chemotherapy, and the advent of interventional endovascular techniques has augmented options that offer a safe, rapid and durable response in terms of symptom relief (Rachapalli and Boucher, 2014). In patients with life-threatening features of SVCS, intravascular stents are particularly useful.

Removal of indwelling catheters and anticoagulation therapy are considerations in patients whose SVCS is due to thrombosis (Wilson et al., 2007). See Table 3.4 for details on therapeutic options.

Table 3.4 Therapeutic options

Therapy	Context	Anticipated Response
Radiotherapy (RT)	• Often used • Majority of tumours sensitive to RT • Tissue diagnosis needed before treatment • Multidisciplinary team planning needed as chemotherapy may also be relevant	• Improvement often apparent within 72 hours but may take a few weeks • Palliative courses typically 1–3 weeks
Systemic chemotherapy	• SVCS in certain malignancies respond very rapidly to chemotherapy alone • Chemotherapy will sometimes be included with RT in the treatment plan	• Courses and responses will vary depending on malignancy
Intravascular stent	• Does not damage tissue that is necessary for diagnosis of cancer • Useful in those with severe symptoms • Useful in mesothelioma • Useful in cases where a thrombosis is associated with an indwelling catheter	• Symptom relief within hours to days
Surgery (surgical bypass grafting)	• Infrequently used • Requires sternotomy or thoracotomy	• System relief rapid

Conclusion

SVCS is clinically striking and may present as a potentially reversible palliative emergency. Most cases are due to a malignancy. In patients with life-threatening features, the placement of an intravascular stent can provide rapid relief of symptoms. In other patients, chemotherapy and radiotherapy are viable treatment options that can relieve the obstructive symptoms in the vast majority of patients.

Malignant Hypercalcaemia

Background

Malignant hypercalcaemia is the most common life-threatening metabolic emergency in patients with cancer (Fowell and Stuart, 2011). It occurs in 20–30% of cancer patients at some point in the course of their illness (Lewis et al., 2011). It is characterised by an abnormally high serum calcium level caused by an underlying cancer. A corrected plasma calcium level above 2.6 mmol/litre defines hypercalcaemia. The most commonly associated cancers include breast, lung, renal and haematological cancers, such as multiple myeloma and lymphoma (Currow and Clark, 2006). It usually occurs in patients with advanced and widespread malignancy and causes a number of distressing symptoms (Minisola et al., 2015). Urgent treatment of hypercalcaemia of malignancy frequently relieves these symptoms and may also impact overall survival (Halfdanarson et al., 2017; Lewis et al., 2011). The attending paramedic should suspect the diagnosis of this potentially reversible life-threatening entity in any cancer patient who is unwell (Fowell and Stuart, 2011).

Impact

The development of hypercalcaemia is a poor prognostic indicator. Median survival after development is three months, although 50% of patients die within thirty days and 80% die within one year (Cherny et al., 2015). Untreated and severe hypercalcaemia is life-threatening, with calcium levels of 4.0 mmol/litre and above causing death in a few days if left untreated (Watson, 2009). In contrast to non-malignant causes of hypercalcaemia, the presentation of hypercalcaemia of malignancy tends to be more florid due to the combination of a more rapid gradient rise in calcium level and a higher absolute calcium level (Sternlicht and Glezerman, 2015). This results in a significant associated morbidity due to multiple burdensome symptoms, reduced function and quality of life.

The acute and chronic treatment options for malignant hypercalcaemia are relatively low burden. An ongoing active malignancy will continue to cause hypercalcaemia (Cherny et al., 2015). Therefore, patients whose prognosis allows and condition warrants will be committed to a form of chronic treatment to control this cancer complication and maintain acceptable symptom control (Fowell and Stuart, 2011). Typical regimes include monthly blood checks and intravenous infusion of bisphosphonate. This can be managed as an outpatient and usually requires a hospital or hospice day-unit attendance. Newer approaches, such as the subcutaneous monoclonal antibody, denosumab, have the advantage of being administered in the community.

Pathophysiology

Three related mechanisms contribute to hypercalcaemia (Cherny et al., 2015). These are summarised in Table 3.5.

All three of these mechanisms occur in malignancy and contribute in varying degrees to the end result of a raised serum calcium concentration. Malignant tumours have the ability to produce abnormal hormones, which can exert their effects distant to the

Table 3.5 Malignant hypercalcaemia mechanisms

Mechanism	Contribution
At the bone level	There is abnormally increased resorption of bone by bone cells called osteoclasts
At the kidney level	The kidneys do not eliminate calcium from the body effectively
At the gut level	There is abnormally enhanced calcium absorption from the gut

primary cancer. This is called a paraneoplastic syndrome. In the case of malignant hypercalcaemia, the tumour often produces an abnormal hormone called PTHrP (Halfdanarson et al., 2017). This hormone exerts its effect at the bone and kidney level resulting in what is known as 'humoral' hypercalcaemia, accounting for 80% of cases (Stewart, 2005). Although it exerts its effect at 'the bone level', because it is a paraneoplastic effect, it does not absolutely require the presence of bone metastases for it to occur. This is important to know because some people mistakenly think bone metastases have to be present for malignant hypercalcaemia to occur. In fact, humoral hypercalcaemia more typically occurs with non-metastatic cancers of renal, ovarian, breast, endometrial or squamous cell origin (Stewart, 2005). Osteolytic bone metastases take effect at the bone and kidney level also and account for 20% of cases. It is most frequently encountered in multiple myeloma and metastatic breast cancer (Sternlicht and Glezerman, 2015). Less than 1% of cases are related to vitamin D metabolism at the gut level and these are usually associated with lymphomas (Sternlicht and Glezerman, 2015).

How Do I Recognise It?

It can be difficult to recognise malignant hypercalcaemia because symptoms and signs may be vague and may mimic several other conditions, including progression of the underlying cancer (Cherny et al., 2015). A high index of suspicion is therefore required, taking into account the WHY framework, risk factors for malignant hypercalcaemia, in combination with a thorough history and relevant examination.

Step 1. Identify the presence of risk factors and exacerbating factors.

- Commonly associated malignancies:
  - Humoral hypercalcaemia is frequently associated with:
    - renal cancer
    - ovarian cancer
    - breast cancer
    - lymphoma
    - squamous cell carcinoma.

- ◆ Local osteolytic hypercalcaemia is frequently associated with:
  - ▸ breast cancer
  - ▸ multiple myeloma
  - ▸ cancers with widespread skeletal involvement.
- ▪ Certain medications can cause or worsen hypercalcaemia (thiazide diuretics, lithium, calcium, over-the-counter antacids, vitamin D) (Stewart, 2005).
- ▪ A previous episode of acute malignant hypercalcaemia places the patient at risk of recurrence.

Step 2. Targeted history and examination.

- ▪ The clinical features of hypercalcaemia of malignancy can be broadly considered using the mnemonic *stones, bones, groans, moans and psychiatric overtones* (Table 3.6).

Table 3.6 Manifestations of hypercalcaemia

Manifestation	Definition
Stones	● Kidney stones are consistent with chronic hypercalcaemia as opposed to acute malignant hypercalcaemia. ● Kidney failure may be a complication.
Bones	● Refers to bone and soft-tissue complications of hypercalcaemia. In the case of malignant hypercalcaemia, may be caused by increased bone turnover due to osteoclast bone cell activation, bone metastases, bone fracture, arthritis, myopathy.
Groans	● Refers to gastrointestinal complications of anorexia, nausea, vomiting, constipation, ileus and, less commonly, peptic ulcer disease or pancreatitis.
Moans	● Refers to general malaise, fatigue, lethargy.
Psychiatric overtones	● Refers to the effects on the central nervous system. Symptoms include fatigue, lethargy, confusion, mental sluggishness, depression, delirium, psychosis, ataxia, seizures, coma.

Pattern Recognition

Hypercalcaemia of malignancy often presents with markedly elevated calcium levels and a rapid rate of increase. It is therefore usually significantly symptomatic (Mirrakhimov, 2015).

Most patients initially develop malaise and lethargy. This is followed by thirst, nausea and constipation before neurological and cardiological features appear. The heart manifestations include bradycardias and dysrhythmias, so an ECG and appropriate cardiac supportive resuscitation may be necessary. There are no characteristic diagnostic features on clinical examination, but it is reasonable to specifically include an assessment of the following:

- Consciousness and cognition (Glasgow coma score, mini-mental test)
- Hydration status (assessing for reduced tissue turgor, hypotension, tachycardia, reduced urine output)
- Cardiovascular status (pulse assessment for bradycardia or other dysrhythmias)
- Gastrointestinal status (constipation is common and obstruction of the intestine due to paralysis of the intestinal muscles, known as paralytic ileus, is possible, so an abdominal examination for distension and auscultation for bowel sounds should be performed).

All symptomatic patients with malignancy should have their serum calcium measured if treatment is likely to be appropriate (Cherny et al., 2015).

Management

As a first responder paramedic, it is unlikely that a blood result will be available to guide the diagnosis, and so the management plan will need to be led by the severity of clinical manifestation and/or anticipated rate of progression. Emergency admission to hospital is required for people with severe hypercalcaemia (>3.5 mmol/litre) or who are severely symptomatic (Minisola et al., 2015).

When malignant hypercalcaemia is clinically suspected, decisions need to be made regarding how best to manage the palliative emergency. Key aspects to consider concerning treatment are shown in Table 3.7.

When treatment is appropriate and desired:

1. Undertake a time-critical transfer to nearest emergency department if the following time-critical features are present, and provide patient management en route and an alert/information call:
   a. major airway, breathing, circulation problems
   b. such as may be as a consequence of hypercalcaemia-induced coma, heart block or cardiac arrhythmia.

2. In the absence of the above time-critical features, suspected malignant hypercalcaemia may still represent an emergency in cases of severe (>3.5 mmol/litre) hypercalcaemia, or in those who experience a rapid rise in serum calcium to more moderate levels, but who have changes in sensorium (e.g. lethargy, stupor). Depending on the symptom severity, transfer to an emergency department may be warranted, or to a specialist unit if advised by an expert team such as the oncology or specialist palliative care teams.

Table 3.7 Relevant considerations for treatment of suspected hypercalcaemia

Context and Considerations	Potential Actions and Outcomes
Natural history and prognosis of disease prior to emergency	• If prognosis is measured in hours to days prior to onset of this problem, then the focus is on symptom control and no interventions to reduce calcium are necessary. • It may be reasonable for those with a prognosis of a number of days and experiencing burdensome symptoms to consider gentle parenteral hydration +/– calcitonin. • Patients with prognoses of weeks, months or years prior to onset of this problem should, in addition to symptom control, be investigated and treated for suspected malignant hypercalcaemia. *Because the symptoms of hypercalcaemia can be distressing and are likely to respond to treatment, pursuing the diagnosis should be seriously considered even for those with limited overall prognosis.
Performance status and general condition of patient	• Consider how treatment of malignant hypercalcaemia may preserve or improve the performance status of the patient. • Does the general condition of the patient permit transfer to a hospital, phlebotomy and general medical work-up? Treatment options are of a low-level invasiveness and are generally well-tolerated.
Patient and family wishes	• Do patient and family desire the anticipated treatment and have they sufficient information to make an informed decision (refer to 'Impact of Malignant Hypercalcaemia' section above)? • Check the patient's capacity for decision making. • Check if an Advance Care Directive specifically addresses this circumstance.
Burden versus benefit treatment	• Burden of treatment – generally well tolerated but potential side effects include flu-like symptoms and site reactions with bisphosphonate infusions, risk of osteonecrosis jaw with bisphosphonates and denosumab, risk of nephrotoxicity with bisphosphonates, risk of low calcium level with denosumab, steroid side effects. • Potential benefits include resolution of burdensome hypercalcaemia symptoms (see Table 3.6) and better survival benefit conferred when treated rather than untreated.
Will treatment improve quality of life?	• What would treatment actually change for the patient? How much value does the patient place on that change? This is very individual.

3. Cases of mild hypercalcaemia (<2.6 mmol/litre) and asymptomatic or mildly symptomatic patients do not require immediate treatment, but a follow-up with the patient's usual physician should be arranged for review and planned admission for treatment.

In-Hospital Treatment

A definitive diagnosis can only be made by biochemical investigation. The biochemical severity of hypercalcaemia may be classified according to the total adjusted serum calcium level (Table 3.8).

The type of treatment and timing of administration should be guided by the clinical manifestations, not just the blood result (Minisola et al., 2015).

Rehydration followed by the administration of calcium-lowering agents is the mainstay of treatment (see Table 3.9).

Haemodialysis may be considered as a treatment option in cases of treatment failure or life-threatening situations. Control or cure of the underlying malignancy is the most definitive treatment of all (Minisola et al., 2015).

Table 3.8 Hypercalcaemia severity stratified by total adjusted serum calcium (mmol/litre)

Hypercalcaemia Severity	Total Adjusted Serum Calcium (mmol/litre)
Mild	2.6–2.9
Moderate	3.0–3.4
Severe	>3.5

Metastatic Spinal Cord Compression

Background

Metastatic Spinal Cord Compression (MSCC) is a cancer-related medical emergency involving pressure on the spinal cord or the nerve roots in the cauda equina that eventually leads to irreversible neurological damage if untreated (Loblaw et al., 2012; Prasad and Schiff, 2005). MSCC represents a time-sensitive emergency; therefore, early identification and transfer for treatment is key to ensuring the best functional outcome for patients. It occurs in up to 6% of patients with cancer at some point throughout their illness (Halfdanarson et al., 2017) and between five and ten in every two hundred patients with advanced cancer will develop MSCC within the last two years of life (Al-Qurainy and Collis, 2016). While most patients diagnosed with MSCC have an established diagnosis of cancer, it is important to bear in mind that the condition may be the presenting feature of new cancers in up to 25% of cases (Levack et al., 2002).

Table 3.9 Treatment of hypercalcaemia of malignancy

Intervention	Regimen	Onset	Duration of Effect	Comment
*Normal saline	2–4 litres per day	Immediate	2–3 days	Infusion rate should be adapted for cardiovascular state of patient
IV bisphosphonate	e.g. zoledronic acid infused over 15 minutes	48–96 hours	3–4 weeks	Needs to be dose adjusted in renal impairment Risk of nephrotoxicity and jaw osteonecrosis
Calcitonin	4–8 units/kg SC every 6–12 hours	4–6 hours	Up to 3 days	A fast acting but temporary holding measure
Corticosteroids	Prednisone 60 mg/day PO; hydrocortisone 100mg every 6 hours IV	7 days	Unclear, perhaps 1–2 weeks	Role is primarily in lymphoma, myeloma
Denosumab	E.g. 60–120 mg weekly SC for 4 weeks, then every 4 weeks but advice on regimes differs	7–10 days	3–4 months	Can cause severe hypoglycaemia

*Isotonic saline at an initial rate of 200–300 mL/hour for volume expansion, then adjusted to maintain urine output 100–150 mL/hour. However, this recommendation depends on multiple factors that must be taken into consideration: severity of hypercalcaemia, age of patient, comorbid conditions, particularly cardiac or renal disease. Fluid replacement must therefore be individualised and based on clinical assessment. An additional challenge for the paramedic at the scene is that there will be no immediately available on-site blood confirmation of hypercalcaemia. Clinical assessment of hydration status as per usual protocol is necessary.

(Minisola, 2015)

MSCC may occur with any cancer, but the most commonly associated malignancies include breast, lung, prostate and renal cancer (Longo et al., 2017). The haematological malignancies, such as multiple myeloma and lymphoma, have a high cancer-specific incidence. Compression of the cord most commonly affects the thoracic spine (60%), followed by lumbar (25%) and cervical segments (15%) (Longo et al., 2017). Multiple levels of compression are discovered in up to a third of cases, hence the recommendation to image the whole spine when performing diagnostic work-up (Al-Qurainy and Collis, 2016).

Treatments that may be considered for the management of MSCC include analgesia, steroids, radiotherapy, surgery and occasionally chemotherapy. The clinical aims of treatment are to preserve or regain motor and sensory function, continence and for pain control. Early recognition coupled with rapid referral pathways and treatment is required.

Impact

Paramedics play a key role in the front-line decision making and management of this potentially reversible emergency. The consequences of a missed diagnosis or delay to treatment are life-altering and the presence of a life-limiting or advanced cancer does not minimise the impact. Understanding and communicating the impact of the condition and implications of the relevant management options underpins informed shared decision making. Much of the literature on the benefits of palliative care includes the prevention of hospital admissions, emergency department attendances and keeping people at home.

But keeping the patient at home 'at all costs' may in fact be too high a price to pay. Patients and families may be very willing to 'trade-off' the burden of an emergency department attendance if they felt there was a reasonable chance of preventing paraplegia or permanent incontinence.

Untreated MSCC results in progressive paralysis, sensory loss, pain and incontinence and is associated with a prognosis of one month (Loblaw et al., 2012). Timely MSCC treatment in appropriate patients results in better outcomes overall (Al-Qurainy and Collis, 2016; Longo et al., 2017; White et al., 2008). Walking ability before treatment is the strongest predictor of walking ability after treatment (Figure 3.4). Retaining walking ability is associated with a longer survival. Survival in patients who develop a MSCC in the context of multiple spinal metastases is generally less than six months, but may be more if walking ability is retained (Longo et al., 2017). For those who have established paraplegia for over 24 hours before getting to treatment, life expectancy is more likely in the range of weeks (Al-Qurainy and Collis, 2016).

Figure 3.5 shows statistics and research findings which emphasise how important a timely diagnosis is, before the onset of motor loss or sphincter disturbance.

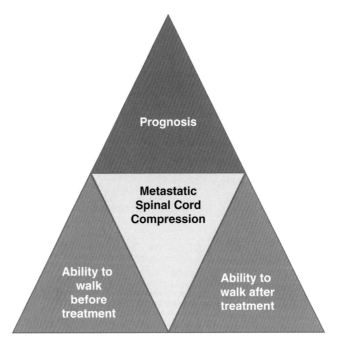

Figure 3.4   Walking ability and MSCC

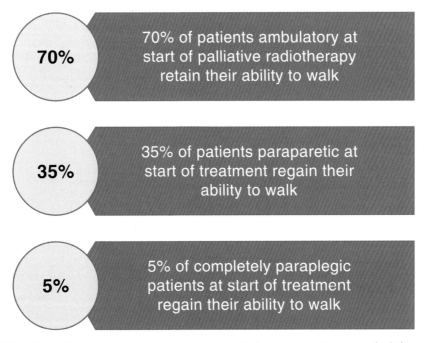

70%   70% of patients ambulatory at start of palliative radiotherapy retain their ability to walk

35%   35% of patients paraparetic at start of treatment regain their ability to walk

5%   5% of completely paraplegic patients at start of treatment regain their ability to walk

Figure 3.5   Statistics concerning palliative radiotherapy patients and ability to walk
Source: Adapted from Falk and Fallon, 1997; Schrijvers, 2011

Over 300 patients with MSCC were interviewed periodically following a diagnosis of cord compression as part of the Scottish Cord Compression Study (Levack, 2010). Key findings from this study were:

- Those unable to walk at diagnosis were significantly more likely to live the remainder of their lives in institutional care.

- Loss of mobility and continence at the time of diagnosis was unlikely to be regained after treatment.

- Uncontrolled pain remained a significant feature for almost half of those affected even one month later.

- Quality of life was reduced for those with poorer performance status.

Other risks associated with immobility become relevant for paraplegic or quadriplegic patients, such as deep vein thrombosis, pressure sores and recurrent infections (Watson et al., 2009). These events compound morbidity and influence mortality. Few studies have examined the impact on carer wellbeing, but experience would suggest it is significant.

Pathophysiology

MSCC is caused by one of three mechanisms:

1. metastases to the vertebral spine causing collapse and compression (causes 85% of MSCC, see Figure 3.6) (Al-Qurainy and Collis, 2016; Bucholtz, 1999)

2. local tumour extending into the spinal cord (Bucholtz, 1999; Savage et al., 2014)

3. deposition of cancer cells directly into the spinal cord (Al-Qurainy and Collis, 2016; Bucholtz, 1999).

The resultant pressure on the spinal cord eventually causes tissue necrosis leading to irreversible nerve damage if untreated.

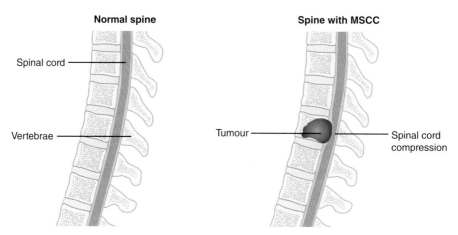

Figure 3.6 Acute cord compression due to metastatic cancer to a vertebral body

Source: This image was produced by Macmillan Cancer Support and is reused with permission

How Do I Recognise It?

It can be difficult to recognise MSCC as evidenced by the fact that 60–85% of patients have the late and often irreversible sign of limb weakness at the time of diagnosis (Al-Qurainy and Collis, 2016). A high index of suspicion is therefore required, taking into account the risk factors for MSCC in combination with a thorough history and targeted examination.

Step 1. Identify patients at risk:

- unknown cancer but clinical features present
- known cancer with back pain and/or other clinical features
- high risk cancers, such as breast, lung, prostate, renal and haematological, with back pain and/or other clinical features
- known spinal metastatic disease or widespread malignancy with back pain and/or other clinical features.

Step 2. Targeted history and examination to identify red flag symptoms:

- The four cardinal domains of MSCC can be considered using the acronym PAMS (Avery and Avery, 2008):

  Pain: a painful back problem

  Autonomic dysfunction: an evacuation problem

  Motor deficits: a movement problem

  Sensory deficits: a feeling problem.

Early Manifestation – Back Pain

Back pain is the most common initial presenting feature of MSCC, occurring in 90% of cases (Lewis et al., 2011). But back pain is common, and differentiating simple back pain or the pain of spinal metastases from the pain of MSCC can be difficult (Al-Qurainy and Collis, 2016; Savage et al., 2014). Spinal metastases are common in cancer, but they only cause MSCC when they extend from the bone to the epidural space and narrow the spinal canal (Longo et al., 2017). UK NICE guidance provides a list of pain characteristics to help identify suspicious spinal pain (red flags) and stratify urgency of response.

Box 1: Characteristics of suggestive spinal metastases

- Pain in the middle (thoracic) or upper (cervical) spine
- Severe unremitting lower spinal pain
- Spinal pain aggravated by straining, coughing or sneezing
- Localised spinal tenderness
- Nocturnal pain preventing sleep.

NICE recommend contacting a designated MSCC coordinator urgently (within 24 hours) to discuss care of patients with cancer and above pain features.

> ## Box 2: Additional features that heighten concern for MSCC requiring emergency transfer
>
> - Neurological symptoms such as radicular pain, limb weakness, difficulty in walking, sensory loss, and bladder or bowel dysfunction
> - Neurological signs of spinal cord or cauda equina compression.
>
> NICE recommend contacting a designated MSCC coordinator immediately to discuss care of patients with cancer and above features. Consider it an oncological emergency.

Additionally, the neoplastic process can disrupt the structural integrity of the spine leading to spinal instability. This has implications for how an associated MSCC is treated. For example, patients with mechanically unstable tumour-related spinal fracture require surgical stabilisation of the spine prior to radiotherapy in order to relieve pain and attain adequate functional outcome. Identification of risk of spinal instability in the context of MSCC is therefore an important clinical endeavour and every patient with pain caused by movement should be considered unstable until proven otherwise.

> ## Box 3: Characteristics of spinal instability
>
> - Movement-related spinal pain
> - Symptomatic or progressive deformity
> - Neural compromise under physiological load.

The back pain associated with MSCC worsens over time and often precedes neurological findings by weeks to months, although a much more acute presentation is also possible. Localised aching or gnawing spinal pain and tenderness on percussion over the affected site may be accompanied by symptoms of nerve root irritation causing radicular pain. This is a girdle-like pain and patients may describe it as a 'band' or like a 'belt tightening' if affecting thoracic or lumbar spine (Al-Qurainy and Collis, 2016). Pain may be worse on lying down and may wake patients from sleep. The WHO pain ladder guides appropriate pain management (see Figure 4.1 in Chapter 4 – Symptom Management).

Steroid therapy also has a role in pain control.

> ### PATIENTS MAY SAY
> - My back pain has increased and it's waking me at night.
> - Descriptors such as gnawing or aching are often used, or sharp radicular pain.

- I need more break-through pain medications than usual.
- My pain moves around my side(s).
- It's like a band or belt squeezing me.
- It gets worse when I go to the toilet, cough, sneeze, lie down.
- It's relieved when I stand up.

ASK THE PATIENT

A pain assessment framework such as SOCRATES should be used to elicit a full history. This will help identify the pain characteristics of spinal metastases (Box 1), as well as associated features that would heighten concern for MSCC (Box 2).

SOCRATES

- **S**ite – where is the pain?
- **O**nset – time of onset? Was this sudden or gradual?
- **C**haracter – what is the pain like?
- **R**adiation – does it radiate anywhere?
- **A**ssociations – are there any other symptoms or signs associated with the pain?
- **T**ime course – does the pain follow any pattern?
- **E**xacerbating/relieving factors – is there anything which changes the pain?
- **S**everity – how bad is the pain?

Late Manifestation – Autonomic Dysfunction

Autonomic dysfunction is usually a late consequence of MSCC. It presents with bowel and bladder problems such as urinary retention, urinary or faecal incontinence or constipation. As the assessing paramedic, you may have to directly ask about these symptoms as patients may not appreciate the relevance of continence to back pain. Constipation appears to be the most common bowel symptom in MSCC (Levack et al., 2002). It is worth noting the importance of direct questioning because a type of compression below the first lumbar spine, known as cauda equina syndrome, may present with bowel and bladder dysfunction in the absence of pain or motor loss – it may be the first feature to alert you to MSCC in this cohort (Al-Qurainy and Collis, 2016). Other possible autonomic symptoms include dizziness or syncope due to hypotension or bradycardia, cold, shivering and drowsiness due to hypothermia, or abdominal pain or distension due to ileus. Such features require appropriate supportive resuscitation measures.

PATIENTS MAY SAY

- Nothing at all.
- My bowels/bladder are leaking.
- I'm constipated.
- I'm having difficulty passing urine – dribbling, stopping and starting, passing small amounts.

ASK THE PATIENT

- Are you able to open your bowels and pass urine normally?
- Have you had any accidents where your bowels have opened or you have passed urine without warning?

Immediate to Late Manifestation – Motor Deficits

Limb weakness affects 60–85% of patients with MSCC at time of diagnosis (Abrahm et al., 2008). This makes weakness the second most common presenting feature of MSCC after back pain. The priority is to get the patient to treatment with the least amount of established neurological deficit, but unfortunately up to 70% of patients are unable to walk at time of presentation. This confers a negative outcome for the patient (see Figures 3.4 and 3.5). Progressive functional impairment over weeks, days or hours should be sought by the assessing paramedic. Neurological examination may reveal motor neurone signs related to the level of cord compression.

PATIENTS MAY SAY

- My legs feel heavy.
- My legs won't carry me up the stairs.
- I find it difficult to stand up.
- My legs give way from under me.
- I'm clumsy – balance is off, falling, not able to grip things as usual.

ASK THE PATIENT

- Has your walking been unsteady or changed recently?
- Do your legs 'give way' from under you?
- Have you had difficulty standing or transferring from bed to chair?
- Have you had falls lately?

Less Common Manifestation – Sensory Deficits

Sensory symptoms are less common and may be present before sensory signs emerge emphasising the importance of good history taking. More than 50% of patients will present with sensory changes. Paraesthesia, reduced sensation or numbness of fingers or toes may then be described as extending upwards as symptoms progress. Examination may reveal a circumferential boundary below which there is a loss of sensation, known as a 'sensory level'. Reduced sensation in the perineal, posterior thigh and buttock area or 'saddle distribution' is in keeping with cauda equina syndrome. A combination of rapid-onset sensory and motor symptoms should raise a high index of suspicion for MSCC (Al-Qurainy and Collis, 2016).

PATIENTS MAY SAY

- My legs/hands/arms feel numb or cold or like 'pins and needles'.
- My legs/hands/arms feel 'funny' (sensory changes can be difficult to describe).

ASK THE PATIENT

- Have you reduced awareness of passing urine or bowel movement?
- Have you any unusual or reduced sensations in your arms or legs? Ask specifically about pins and needles, numbness, coldness if not volunteered.

Early diagnosis can be challenging because the classical features of cord compression, limb weakness and sensory loss, bowel and bladder dysfunction, occur late in the presentation. It is worth noting that physical signs may be absent in early MSCC and therefore should not be depended on for the condition to be clinically suspected.

Management

The goals of treatment for patients with MSCC include pain control, avoidance of complications, and the preservation or improvement of neurological function and spinal mechanical stability using treatments appropriate to the patient's burden of disease, life expectancy, values and preferences, and goals for care (Lawton et al., 2019). Consider the information in Table 3.10 when deciding on treatment for a patient with MSCC.

When treatment is appropriate and desired:

1. Undertake a time-critical transfer to nearest emergency department if the following time critical features present, and provide patient management en route:

    a. major airway, breathing, circulation, disability (ABCD) problems (such as may present with spinal shock)

    b. neurological signs of spinal cord or cauda equina compression.

Table 3.10 Relevant considerations for treatment of MSCC

Context and Considerations	Potential Actions and Outcomes
Natural history and prognosis of disease prior to emergency	● Prognosis measured in hours to days, dying patient: further investigations not indicated. Attention to pain control, bowel/bladder control, general care needs. ● Prognosis measured in weeks or months: further investigations likely indicated in addition to symptom control. *Because paralysis and paresis are such devastating complications, and because therapy is well tolerated, pursuing the diagnosis should be seriously considered even for those with limited overall prognosis.*
Performance status and general condition of patient	● Consider how treatment of MSCC may preserve or improve the performance status of the patient (see Figure 3.7). ● Does the general condition of the patient permit transfer to a hospital and at least one fraction of radiotherapy (15 minutes on relatively hard-topped table and able to follow commands)? Diagnostic MRI scan requires patient to remain still and lying for 40 minutes. Analgesia may be used.
Patient and family wishes	● Do patient and family desire the anticipated treatment and have they sufficient information to make an informed decision (refer to 'Impact of MSCC' section above)? ● Check the patient's capacity for decision making. ● Check if an Advance Care Directive specifically addresses this circumstance.
Burden versus benefit treatment	● Radiotherapy: usually between a single fraction to five fractions (delivered over 1–5 days). Improvement begins a few days later but full effect may take 4–6 weeks. Low level of toxicity. ● Surgery: requires 2–3 months recovery time. ● Potential benefits include mobility, continence, pain control and increased survival.
Will treatment improve quality of life?	● What would treatment actually change for the patient? How much value does the patient place on that change? This is very individual.

2. In the absence of the above time-critical features, suspected MSCC remains a medical emergency, but discussion with the regional MSCC coordinator or expert team may direct transfer to a specialist unit. Otherwise proceed to transfer to nearest emergency department.

3. Position supine with neutral spine alignment for patients with severe pain, neurological symptoms or signs of compression (NICE, 2008).

4. Assess and record pain. Offer analgesia. Be guided by the WHO analgesia ladder or local pain management guidelines.

Radiotherapy

- Goals of treatment are prevention of neurological deterioration, improvement of neurological function and pain relief.
- *Good prognosis regime usually involves 5–10 daily fractions.
- **Poor prognosis regime supports a single fraction primarily for pain relief.
- Stereotactic body radiation therapy (SBRT) is considered in certain instances.

Surgery

- Goals of treatment are to decompress the spinal cord and reconstruct and stabilise the spinal column.
- It is the most rapid method for relief of acute compression and considered if there is spinal instability, or single-level tumour.
- Patients whose life expectancy is less than six months are typically not suitable and should be considered for palliative radiotherapy instead.

Chemotherapy

- Chemotherapy may have a role in certain chemo-sensitive malignancies such as lymphoma and small cell lung cancer

Figure 3.7 Benefits and goals of radiotherapy/surgery/chemotherapy

*Good prognosis = Ambulatory, or immobility less than 24 hours and life expectancy greater than six months

**Poor prognosis = Established paraplegia more than 24 hours, poor performance status and life expectancy less than six months

In-Hospital Treatment

To confirm a diagnosis of MSCC, the gold standard investigation is a whole spine MRI scan. This should be performed urgently to facilitate treatment within 24 hours of the suspected diagnosis of MSCC (NICE, 2008). Patients typically receive high dose corticosteroids to reduce cord oedema, and thus the degree of compression, and to aid pain control as a temporary measure (NICE 2008).

Once a diagnosis is established, treatment options include any combination of radiotherapy, surgery and chemotherapy (Figure 3.7). Therapy depends on several factors including the type of cancer, location of tumour, speed of symptom onset, pre-treatment function and life expectancy. In view of these factors palliative radiotherapy is the most common treatment line.

Holistic Care

The aim should be to focus on person-centred goals of care and optimising quality of life. A multidisciplinary approach has much to offer and rehabilitation options should consider a patient's preferred place of care.

Neutropenic Sepsis

Background

Neutropenic sepsis is a serious, life-threatening complication of systemic anti-cancer therapy (SACT) and bone marrow dysfunction. It has significant associated morbidity and mortality rates. The greatest risk of developing neutropenic sepsis is with cytotoxic chemotherapy, although radiotherapy, direct tumour effects and non-cancer causes can occasionally be responsible. The focus in this chapter is on neutropenic sepsis as a complication of SACT. Definitions on what constitutes neutropenic sepsis in this context also vary and exact protocols may differ slightly depending on your local trust: Please familiarise yourself with local trust guidance and also refer to JRCALC guidelines. For the purpose of this chapter, we will adhere to the National Institute for Health and Care Excellence (NICE) guidance for neutropenic sepsis management and recognise neutropenic sepsis as that occurring in:

> patients having anticancer treatment whose neutrophil count is 0.5 x 109 per litre or lower and who have either:
>
> - a temperature higher than 38°C or/and
> - other signs or symptoms consistent with clinically significant sepsis.
>
> (NICE, 2012)

The terms 'neutropenic sepsis', 'febrile neutropenia' and 'neutropenic fever syndromes' are often used interchangeably in practice. NICE guidance refers to these entities under 'neutropenic sepsis'. The same approach applies in this chapter. Sepsis

Table 3.11 Systemic manifestations of sepsis

Domains	Clinical Indicators of Sepsis
General	<ul><li>Temperature >38.3°C/>38°C for 1 hour or <36°C</li><li>Tachycardia</li><li>Tachypnoea</li><li>Altered mental state</li><li>Significant fluid retention</li><li>High plasma glucose (in absence of diabetes)</li></ul>
Inflammatory	<ul><li>High or low white blood cell count (less relevant in neutropenic sepsis)</li><li>Raised serum inflammatory markers (C-reactive protein, procalcitonin)</li></ul>
Haemodynamic	<ul><li>Arterial hypotension</li></ul>
Organ dysfunction*	<ul><li>Hypoxaemia</li><li>Reduced urine output</li><li>Blood tests demonstrating organ dysfunction (creatinine, platelets, INR, bilirubin)</li><li>Ileus (absent bowel sounds)</li></ul>
Tissue perfusion*	<ul><li>Decreased capillary refill or mottling</li><li>High lactate level</li></ul>

Consistent with severe sepsis

(Levy et al., 2003; Rhodes et al., 2017)

is defined as the presence (probable or documented) of infection together with some of the systemic manifestations of infection. Sepsis is considered severe when there is also sepsis-induced organ dysfunction or tissue hypoperfusion (Levy et al., 2003; Rhodes et al., 2017). Refer to Table 3.11 for the systemic manifestations of sepsis.

Sepsis in general is a time-dependent medical emergency that demands early resuscitation with urgent antibiotics, and neutropenic sepsis is viewed in the same light (Dellinger et al., 2013; Rhodes et al., 2017). It is essential to consider whether a septic patient may also be neutropenic and thus at high risk of complications (Welsh and Strauss, 2012). A target one hour 'door-to-needle' time for the administration of first dose antibiotics on arrival to hospital continues to be reflected in many trust's local neutropenic sepsis protocols. This practice has been transposed from the international Surviving Sepsis Campaign's gold standard and reflects a pragmatic approach to ensuring rapid treatment in a potentially fatal condition (Dellinger et al., 2013). All cases of suspected neutropenic sepsis should be considered a medical emergency that requires immediate hospital investigation and treatment (Talbot et al., 2017).

The incidence of neutropenic sepsis is unclear but the number of deaths from this cancer-treatment complication is increasing, very likely due to the increase in the amount of chemotherapy being administered (National Chemotherapy Advisory Group, NCAG, 2009). Systemic anti-cancer therapy (SACT) is most frequently administered in an outpatient or day-case setting, therefore most episodes of neutropenic sepsis will present in the community (NICE, 2012). Consequently, it is most likely that this complication will be increasingly encountered by paramedics attending emergencies in the community.

Additionally, it is important to appreciate that this emergency does not relate solely to patients receiving treatment with curative intent, but that it can occur in patients with advanced disease who are in receipt of palliative anti-cancer therapy (Lalami and Klastersky, 2017). The timeline of chemotherapy use in cancer patients has elongated over the last decade due to advances in novel, high-efficacy anti-cancer therapeutic agents (Lee et al., 2015). Palliative anti-cancer developments, coupled with the early integration of palliative care in cancer care, creates a situation whereby paramedics are increasingly likely to be confronted with this medical emergency in a community palliative setting.

Impact

Neutropenic sepsis is common, resulting in hundreds of hospital admissions every month and potentially causing the deaths of over 1 in 500 people diagnosed with cancer (NICE, 2012). Considerable concern surrounding serious shortcomings in neutropenic sepsis management in the United Kingdom arose in 2008 (Mort et al., 2008).

It was determined that avoidable patient deaths following chemotherapy were occurring as a result of these shortcomings. Evidence-based guidelines were subsequently developed to improve the quality of care and reduce avoidable poor outcomes (NCAG, 2009; NICE, 2012). Neutropenic sepsis remains associated with substantial morbidity, mortality and costs despite therapeutic advances over the last decades (Klastersky et al., 2000; Smith et al., 2015). Mortality rates range from 2–21% and tend to be higher in those with comorbidities (Lalami and Klastersky, 2017). It may result in significant physical, social and emotional consequences for patients receiving SACT (Warnock, 2016). Cancer treatment implications include delays or dose reductions in subsequent chemotherapy cycles, chemotherapy discontinuation, or switching to alternative agents (Lalami and Klastersky, 2017). Any of these may jeopardise optimal disease outcomes. In certain circumstances, measures to reduce the risk of neutropenic sepsis may be appropriate, such as prophylactic antibiotics or bone marrow stimulant.

Pathophysiology

Neutrophils are known as the 'innate soldiers of the immune system' and are the most prolific and the first to respond of all the immune cells. When functioning normally, they move towards microbes, usually bacteria or fungi, and ingest and kill them. Patients who are neutropenic therefore have a reduced ability to fight infection and are at increased risk of developing neutropenic sepsis (Lewis et al., 2011). SACT causes this neutropenia as an unwanted by-product of the mechanism required for it to do its job of killing neoplastic stem cells. The DNA damage required to kill neoplastic cells also particularly affects the more rapidly dividing normal tissues in our bodies such as:

- **Hair follicles** – resulting in alopecia
- **Mucosal linings** – resulting in mucositis
- **Bone marrow cells** – resulting in anaemia, thrombocytopenia and neutropenia.

In addition to causing neutropenia that makes the patient vulnerable to invasive infection, SACT associated mucositis may also act as a port-of-entry for 'normal' gut bacteria to enter the blood stream causing infective or inflammatory reactions.

The 3 Rs – Recognition, Resuscitation, Referral

Unfortunately, there is insufficient evidence to recommend which symptoms and signs experienced by patients in the community predict neutropenic sepsis (NICE 2012). There is wide variation in how neutropenic sepsis can present, ranging from uncomplicated fever, right up to septic shock without fever (NICE, 2012), so a high index of suspicion is crucial. A contributing factor to this heterogeneity is the altered immune response due to the low number of immune cells or neutrophils. Some studies have shown that confused mental state, chills, or feeling or looking unwell correlated with a poor outcome. However, the absence of these symptoms and signs does not rule out a poor outcome either and there is concern about how generalisable the findings of these studies actually are. Notably, up to 50% of cases of neutropenic sepsis will not have an obvious focus of infection, and not all patients will have a fever (van der Velden et al., 2014). In the pre-hospital setting, there is the additional challenge of not having blood results such as neutrophil counts and other relevant sepsis markers such as lactate and C-reactive protein (see Table 3.11). Given the wide variation in presentation and potential for absence or attenuation of classic signs of sepsis, the following points are important for the assessing paramedic:

1. Always use clinical judgement.
2. Incorporate the WHY framework into the assessment.
3. Take a good history including assessment for risk factors and perform a targeted examination looking for a focus of infection and systemic signs of sepsis (Table 3.11).
4. Have a high index of clinical suspicion when patients have recently received SACT and present themselves as feeling unwell.

More research is needed in this area, but until such evidence is available, NICE guidance is very clear that cancer patients on SACT who become unwell at home, with or without a fever, should be urgently assessed in hospital to allow a rapid diagnosis to be made.

Many patients will have received a chemotherapy alert card from their oncology centre, and it is always worth enquiring about it, as it may contain relevant information that will guide your pre-hospital assessment.

How Do I Recognise It?

When Is It Likely to Happen?

Typically the neutrophil count falls to its lowest level five to ten days after the receipt of chemotherapy, and may take between two and four weeks to recover (Holmes et al., 2002; Lewis et al., 2011). This is relevant because the risks of mortality and other adverse clinical outcomes increase as the absolute neutrophil count falls. Therefore, these are high risk times for the development of neutropenic sepsis. There is a tendency for neutropenic sepsis to occur more commonly in the first two cycles of treatment (Lyman et al., 2005). While novel biological agents generally have a lower rate of neutropenia than cytotoxic chemotherapy, such problems can still occur. More recently, receipt of SACT in the preceding six weeks has been advocated for use in emergency triage departments to identify patients at risk of being neutropenic.

ASK THE PATIENT

- What type of chemotherapy/radiotherapy/immunotherapy are you on?
- When did you last receive chemotherapy?
- What cycle of chemotherapy are you on?

In Whom Is It Likely to Happen?

Risk factors for neutropenic sepsis can include advanced age, poor performance status, poor nutritional status, comorbidities, underlying haematological malignancy and type or intensity of chemotherapy (Lyman et al., 2005). Other points to note include a history of prior neutropenic sepsis and prophylaxis use, suggesting either an 'at-risk patient' or 'at-risk therapy'.

ASK THE PATIENT

- What type of cancer are you being treated for?
- Do you take scheduled antibiotics with your chemotherapy regime?
- Do you receive injections to boost your blood cell count with your chemotherapy regime?
- What other medical conditions do you have?

Clinical History and Examination

It is critical to recognise neutropenic fever early and initiate appropriate antibiotic therapy early in order to prevent progression to sepsis syndrome and possibly death. Given the impaired ability of immunocompromised patients to mount an adequate response to infection, the classic signs and symptoms may be minimal. The predominant sign at diagnosis is fever and there may be localising signs of infection.

CONSIDERATIONS

- Ask about temperature in past 24 hours and measure temperature.
- Screening questions and targeted examination for a source of infection – emphasis on oral cavity, oropharynx, skin, lungs, abdomen, genito-urinary and peri-anal area. All indwelling venous catheters should be examined. Central nervous system infections may present with confusion.
- Ask about general 'flu-like' symptoms.
- Assess for systemic manifestations of sepsis (see Table 3.11).

The initial clinical evaluation should also focus on assessing risk for serious complications. Validated scoring systems assist in this evaluation, such as the Multinational Association of Supportive Care in Cancer (MASCC) score. This evaluation tool identifies nine independent predictive factors which are individually weighted with a differing score. When combined these factors produce a score which is indicative of the likelihood of resolution of neutropenic sepsis without serious medical complications (MASCC, 2019). Mortality varies according to the prognostic index: lower than 5% if the MASCC score is ≥21, but possibly as high as 40% if the MASCC score is <15 (Klastersky et al., 2000).

Resuscitation and Referral

When neutropenic sepsis is suspected, decisions need to be made regarding how best to manage the emergency (Table 3.12).

When treatment is appropriate and desired:

1. If any of the following time-critical features present:
    a. major airway, breathing, circulation (ABC) problems
    b. altered consciousness:
        i. Start correcting ABC problems.
        ii. Undertake a time-critical transfer to nearest emergency department. Provide patient management en route.
        iii. Provide an alert/information call.
2. Manage as per sepsis guidelines.
3. Identify patient alert card and contact oncology unit.
4. Transfer to nearest emergency department or to a specialist unit if advised by a specialist team.

Table 3.12 Relevant considerations for treatment of suspected neutropenic sepsis

Context and Considerations	Potential Actions and Outcomes
Natural history and prognosis of disease prior to emergency	• Prognosis measured in hours to days prior to the onset of this problem, anticipated dying patient. Further investigations not indicated. Attention to palliation of fever, rigors, pain, symptoms of dying patient. • Prognosis measured in weeks or months prior to onset of this problem. Emergency investigation and treatment indicated in addition to symptom control.
Performance status and general condition of patient	• Consider how treatment of neutropenic sepsis may preserve or improve the performance status and survival of the patient. • Does the general condition of the patient permit transfer to a hospital? Unless the patient is actively dying, emergency transfer should be seriously considered.
Patient and family wishes	• Do patient and family desire the anticipated treatment and have they sufficient information to make an informed decision (refer to 'Impact of Neutropenic Sepsis' section above)? • Check the patient's capacity for decision making. • Check if an Advance Care Directive specifically addresses this circumstance.
Burden versus benefit treatment	• Benefits include improved survival rates, less interruption of life-prolonging and symptom control treatments, improved quality of life, less likely to need intensive care management with prompt treatment. • Burden includes hospital admission, IV antibiotics, may need intensive care treatment, morbidity associated with critical care.
Will treatment improve quality of life?	• What would treatment actually change for the patient? How much value does the patient place on that change?

In-Hospital Treatment

Many trusts now have local policies and protocols that incorporate the evidence-based NICE guidance for the management of neutropenic sepsis (NICE, 2012). Rapid empirical antibiotic administration (often the goal is door-to-needle time of one hour) is a key management step in neutropenic sepsis. Piperacillin/tazobactam in addition to gentamicin is the most frequently used empirical antibiotic combination. Appropriate resuscitation and critical care management should be implemented in conjunction with investigation of the potential source of sepsis and tailored therapy. Risk of sepsis severity is assessed and stratified using tools and helps to guide decisions around aggressiveness of care. Timely and repeated senior medical reviews and management plans are necessary to ensure the best outcome for patients.

Catastrophic Events in Terminal Patients

Background

Catastrophic terminal events lead to the death of the patient within minutes of onset. They are rare yet distressing events. Massive haemorrhage or complete airway obstruction are two such examples. For those patients experiencing a life-threatening event in whom resuscitation or definitive treatment is not appropriate the focus of care should be to minimise the distress of imminent death.

While such catastrophic events are rare, the growing focus on the provision of end of life care in the home means that the potential for these events to occur in this setting is likely to increase (Ubogagu and Harris, 2012). Ideally, the feasibility of managing such an event in the home will have been considered sensitively with the patient's family and appropriate preparatory measures taken for those deemed at risk. Adequate support for family and staff following such an event should also be considered.

Terminal Haemorrhage

Terminal haemorrhage is a rare yet distressing emergency in palliative care and is most common in, although not limited to, the palliative oncology population (Harris and Noble, 2009). It may be considered as 'major bleeding from an artery which is likely to cause death within a period of time that may be as short as minutes' (Harris and Noble, 2009). There is, however, no consensus on a definition and terms such as 'terminal haemorrhage', 'catastrophic bleed' and 'major bleed' are used interchangeably. Reported incidence rates vary from 3–12% but these figures are thought perhaps to over-state the problem in part due to the lack of definition (Ubogagu and Harris, 2012).

A terminal haemorrhage causes a rapid reduction in circulating blood volume and causes include (Cherny et al., 2015):

- Internal factors (erosion of thoracic or abdominal vessels causing haemoptysis or haematemesis or rectal bleeding)
- External factors (rupture of carotid or femoral artery).

Certain tumour and treatment-related factors in addition to systemic factors are associated with an increased risk of terminal or catastrophic bleeding (Figure 3.8).

Patients who have experienced a 'herald' or warning bleed are also at increased risk of progressing to a catastrophic bleed and its occurrence should prompt further risk assessment and appropriate risk modification such as medication rationalisation (e.g. cessation of anticoagulants) or more definitive procedures such as photocoagulation where deemed appropriate.

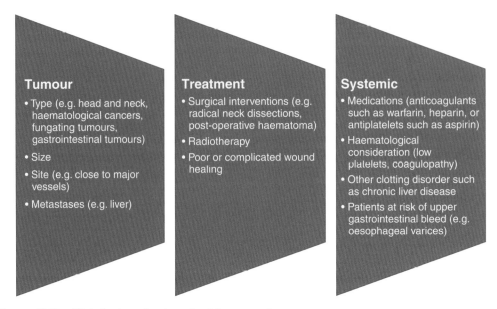

Tumour
- Type (e.g. head and neck, haematological cancers, fungating tumours, gastrointestinal tumours)
- Size
- Site (e.g. close to major vessels)
- Metastases (e.g. liver)

Treatment
- Surgical interventions (e.g. radical neck dissections, post-operative haematoma)
- Radiotherapy
- Poor or complicated wound healing

Systemic
- Medications (anticoagulants such as warfarin, heparin, or antiplatelets such as aspirin)
- Haematological consideration (low platelets, coagulopathy)
- Other clotting disorder such as chronic liver disease
- Patients at risk of upper gastrointestinal bleed (e.g. oesophageal varices)

Figure 3.8   Risk factors for terminal haemorrhage

Preparing for the Event

Certain preparatory measures may take place for palliative care patients with a Do Not Actively Resuscitate Order in place who are also receiving end of life care at home and who have been identified as being at risk of a terminal haemorrhage. Where appropriate, these may include:

- A sensitive yet pragmatic discussion with key family members and care providers in relation to the risk of the event, how to manage it, emergency numbers, and the role of a '999' call in these circumstances.

- Establishment of goals of care, and that resuscitation will not be performed in the event of terminal haemorrhage. This may be included in the patient care plan documentation.

- Ensuring appropriate equipment is available (personal protective equipment, dark towels to reduce distress of the visibility of blood, crisis pack which may contain opioid and anxiolytics) (Harris et al., 2011).

Management of the Event

Arriving at the scene of a haemorrhage that will be fatal in a palliative community context can be a stressful and challenging scenario for paramedics. There is limited time available for active management, so after clarifying goals of care, accepting the constraints of the situation is a key factor in enabling the delivery of reassurance and support to patient and family.

Notably, the current guidance for the management of a terminal haemorrhage in the palliative care setting is based on a limited body of evidence. For guidance on suggested steps to take when managing a terminal haemorrhage see Table 3.13.

Table 3.13 Steps in managing a terminal haemorrhage

Actions	Reason for Action
Staying with the patient	This is the single most important aspect of management. Providing verbal support and concealing the sight of blood with dark towels is a priority. The role of the paramedic is to provide acute support during the immediate distress of the event.
*Crisis packs/ medications	The role of crisis packs is somewhat limited and controversial. In a true rapid terminal event, there is not enough time for these medications to exert a meaningful effect in the setting of a rapidly depleting blood volume. Their use may also detract from staying with the patient, who is likely to die before medication administration. Guidelines recommend these medications be given when practicable. They likely have more of a role when the event is not indeed a true 'terminal' haemorrhage which will be fatal in short minutes, but rather in the event of a slower major haemorrhage which continues for some time before death. NB: The goal of 'crisis medications' is not to hasten death but to reduce awareness and therefore distress. Midazolam is the most commonly used drug and is administered by the most readily available route, most usually at a dose of midazolam 10mg buccal/IV/SC. This may be repeated at 5–10 minute intervals as clinically indicated. Opioids are indicated if there is associated pain and/or dyspnoea.
ABC Aide Memoir	In such a fraught and rapidly changing situation in a patient's home, it is challenging to ground oneself in an approach that is based on staying with a patient in extremis, where medications may have a limited role given the speed of the event. Ubogagu and Harris (2012) have developed a useful algorithm to support the attending healthcare professional (Figure 3.9).

*Supply of anxiolytic (usually midazolam) +/− opioid for the purpose of reducing patient distress and/or pain, and/or dyspnoea.

(Based on Ubogagu and Harris, 2012)

Complete Airway Obstruction

Management of complete airway obstruction requires an individualised approach. The degree of obstruction or narrowing and the rapidity of onset can precipitate a palliative care emergency. While the underlying cause may not be changing quickly, the symptoms of anxiety and dyspnoea can rapidly and significantly escalate affecting patients, families, and healthcare professionals and resulting in a challenging clinical scenario that requires urgent action.

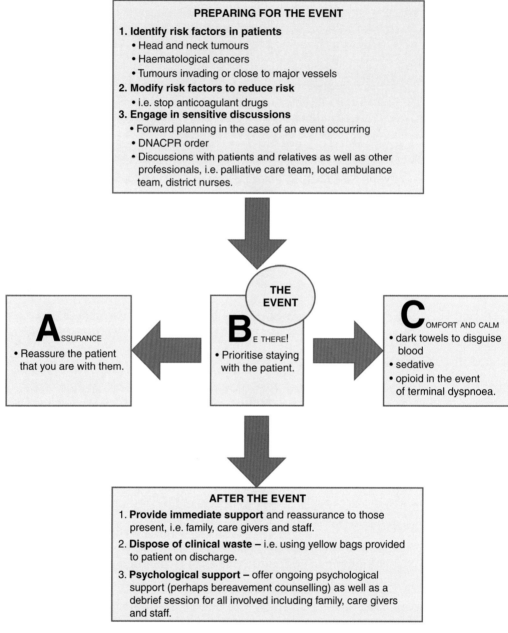

Figure 3.9 ABC algorithm for the management of terminal haemorrhage in the community

Source: Adapted from Ubogagu E and Harris (2012)

Palliative patients who present with stridor (harsh, high-pitched wheezing or vibrating sound that results from turbulent airflow in the upper airways) due to severe tracheal or mainstem obstruction or severe laryngeal oedema and respiratory compromise represent a true medical emergency. Respiratory failure and death are likely outcomes and they require initial stabilisation to secure ventilation and oxygenation, if this is consistent with the goals of care. In these instances, adhere to local protocols/guidelines in relation to the management of a difficult airway.

Reversible factors such as sputum plugging or mechanical blockage or kinking of a tracheostomy tube should be considered, and in certain cases urgent referral for consideration of procedures such as endobronchial stenting, laser or palliative radiotherapy may be warranted.

In some cases however, complete airway obstruction is an anticipated terminal event, and such interventions are inappropriate. Where there is a 'Do Not Actively Resuscitate' order in place and the patient is at home for end of life care, where risk of obstruction is acknowledged and the desire is to manage at home, there is some overlap in the preparation for and management of its consequences and that of the outlined approach for terminal haemorrhage.

Risk factors for complete airway obstruction include:

- Tumours close to major airways such as central lung tumours, head and neck tumours
- Those with signs of partial airway obstruction, such as stridor or refractory wheeze.

These features should prompt consideration of anticipatory planning.

Preparing for the Event

Individualised anticipatory care plans may include:

- A sensitive yet pragmatic discussion with key family members and care providers in relation to risk of event, how to manage, emergency numbers, and the role of a '999' call in these circumstances.
- Establishment of goals of care, and that resuscitation will not be performed in the event of terminal haemorrhage. This may be included in patient care plan documentation.
- Ensuring appropriate equipment available (suction, oxygen, crisis medications as per terminal haemorrhage protocol above).

Managing the Event

A calm reassuring environment is important. Consider sitting the patient upright and providing oxygen/suctioning where appropriate. These measures are less helpful if the patient is sedated. Administer appropriate medications to manage the prominent symptoms of dyspnoea and anxiety. For example, in an opioid-naïve patient, 5 to 10 mg morphine sulphate may be administered intravenously or subcutaneously, repeated every 10 minutes to effect. Sublingual or IV lorazepam may be used for anxiety if tolerated, or more usually if there is a crisis pack in the home, buccal/subcutaneous/intravenous midazolam 5–10 mg. Sedation may be required to relieve distress. An infusion of medications for ongoing symptom control may be necessary and will require the input of a physician to advise.

While the express goal in the event of catastrophic or near catastrophic events may well have been to remain at home, there are instances where community management will not suffice and transfer to a specialist unit for ongoing care may need to be considered. Therefore view all cases and care plans as highly individualised.

Case Studies

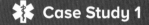 Case Study 1

Marie is a 57-year-old married woman with metastatic breast cancer who lives with her husband John and youngest child Damien who has Down's Syndrome. John has called 999 because Marie's vague symptoms of one week's duration have escalated. Her nausea has progressed to vomiting, which occurs on a background of constipation and increasing fatigue over the last week. She has developed acute confusion this evening with agitation and is frightening Damien. Her medications have been relatively stable over the past number of weeks, although she has been using a non-steroidal anti-inflammatory for generalised bone pains. John is really worried as this is a rapid change in Marie's previously stable disease and he wants her to be brought to hospital.

When you arrive at the house, it is 11 pm. Marie's agitation has settled but she looks quite dehydrated and remains mildly confused.

- What, at this point, is your main differential diagnosis?
- How urgent do you think that Marie's treatment needs to be?

John feels that the situation is calmer and it would be too unsettling for Damien to now go to the emergency department with John and Marie. John is happy to wait until the morning.

- How do you discuss the best course of action with John and what shapes your decision making?

Case Study 2

Thomas is a 67-year-old bachelor with metastatic prostate cancer with extensive bone secondaries. He gave up work 15 years ago due to a back injury on a building site and probably has an alcohol misuse problem. He lives alone in a third-storey flat and mobilises quite well with the aid of a walking stick; he is independent in the activities of daily living. His neighbour Jack has dialled 999 because when he called around for a game of cards, he found Thomas lying on the floor.

When you arrive at the house, Jack has moved Thomas off the floor onto a chair in the kitchen. He has been incontinent of urine and describes severe lower back pain radiating around the right flank.

- What is your primary concern here in terms of pathology?
- What else would you ask about to confirm your suspicions?
- How would you like to manage this situation now that you've formed your opinion?

Thomas refuses to go to hospital. He just wants some pain killers and someone to put him back to bed. He wants everyone to stop bothering him and orders you to leave.

- How do you explain the implications of Thomas' decision to him?
- What else might you try to do to support him?

✳ Case Study 3

Estelle is a 42-year-old woman on chemotherapy for non-small cell lung cancer. She is separated and had been working as a fashion buyer up until the time of her diagnosis. She is on cycle two, day eight of treatment and has just been on the internet looking up treatment side-effects. She has called the emergency services because she has just read about neutropenic sepsis and feels a 'chill'. She thinks she needs to go to hospital.

When you arrive at the house, Estelle answers the door herself and brings you into the kitchen area where she was eating her dinner just before you arrived. She appears well hydrated and her temperature is 37.7°C. She just took a paracetamol 20 minutes before you arrived in case her temperature was increasing. She has a mild dry cough.

- What do you think the likelihood of neutropenic sepsis is in this case?
- Do you have enough evidence to make a management decision?
- Who else might you call to support the decision making?

✳ Case Study 4

Hal is a 71-year-old smoker who is awaiting an appointment in the rapid access lung clinic for investigation of recurrent pneumonia and weight loss. His wife Marian dialled 999 in a panic because Hal developed sudden noisy rasping breathing and is struggling to catch his breath. She has tried a Heimlich manoeuvre in case something had caught in his throat. It hasn't helped.

When you arrive at the house, Hal is in extremis. He is cyanosed, O_2 saturations are 89%, he is tachypnoeic and his face is suffused.

- What do you suspect is happening here?

- What are your first management steps?

Marian is distraught, she thinks Hal is dying.

- How do you explain to her what you think is happening, how it might be treated and the likely success of treatment?

References

Abrahm JL, Banffy MB and Harris MB (2008). Spinal cord compression in patients with advanced metastatic cancer: 'All I care about is walking and living my life'. *JAMA*, 299(8): 937–946.

Al-Qurainy R and Collis E (2016). Metastatic spinal cord compression: diagnosis and management. *BMJ*, 353: i2539.

Avery JD and Avery JA (2008). Malignant spinal cord compression: a hospice emergency. *Home Healthcare Nurse*, 26(8): 457–460.

Bucholtz JD (1999). Metastatic epidural spinal cord compression. *Seminars in Oncology Nursing*, 15(3): 150–159.

Cherny et al. (2015). *Oxford Textbook of Palliative Care Medicine* (5th ed.). Oxford: Oxford University Press.

Currow D and Clark C (2006). *Emergencies in Palliative and Supportive Care*. New York: Oxford University Press.

Dellinger R et al. (2013). Surviving Sepsis Campaign: International guidelines for management of severe sepsis and septic shock, 2012. *Intensive Care Medicine*, 39(2): 165–228.

Donnelly C et al. (2015). Emergency medical services providers' knowledge, attitudes, and experiences responding to patients with end-of-life emergencies (S727). *Journal of Pain and Symptom Management*, 49(2): 421.

Falk S and Fallon M (1997). ABC of palliative care. Emergencies. *BMJ (Clinical research ed.)*, 315(7121): 1525.

Fowell A and Stuart NSA (2011). Emergencies in palliative medicine. *Medicine*, 39(11): 660–663.

Halfdanarson TR, Hogan WJ and Madsen BE (2017). Emergencies in hematology and oncology. *Mayo Clinic Proceedings*, 92(4): 609–641.

Harris DG and Noble SI (2009). Management of terminal hemorrhage in patients with advanced cancer: a systematic literature review. *Journal of Pain and Symptom Management*, 38(6): 913–927.

Harris DG et al. (2011). The use of crisis medication in the management of terminal haemorrhage due to incurable cancer: a qualitative study. *Palliative Medicine*, 25(7): 691–700.

Holmes FA et al. (2002). Comparable efficacy and safety profiles of once-per-cycle pegfilgrastim and daily injection filgrastim in chemotherapy-induced neutropenia: a multicenter dose-finding study in women with breast cancer. *Annals of Oncology*, 13(6): 903–909.

Klastersky J et al. (2000). The Multinational Association for Supportive Care in Cancer risk index: a multinational scoring system for identifying low-risk febrile neutropenic cancer patients. *Journal of Clinical Oncology*, 18(16): 3038.

Lalami Y and Klastersky J (2017). Impact of chemotherapy-induced neutropenia (CIN) and febrile neutropenia (FN) on cancer treatment outcomes: an overview about well-established and recently emerging clinical data. *Critical Reviews in Oncology/Hematology*, 120: 163–179.

Lawton A et al. (2019). Assessment and management of patients with metastatic spinal cord compression: a multidisciplinary review. *Journal of Clinical Oncology*, 37(1): 61–71.

Lee HS et al. (2015). Trends in receiving chemotherapy for advanced cancer patients at the end of life. *BMC Palliative Care*, 14: 4.

Levack P (2010). A13 Survival, function and quality of life after malignant cord compression. *European Journal of Oncology Nursing*, 14: S5–S6.

Levack P et al. (2002). Don't wait for a sensory level – listen to the symptoms: a prospective audit of the delays in diagnosis of malignant cord compression. *Clinical Oncology*, 14(6): 472–480.

Levy MM et al. (2003). 2001 SCCM/ESICM/ACCP/ATS/SIS International Sepsis Definitions Conference. *Intensive Care Medicine*, 29(4): 530–538.

Lewis MA, Hendrickson AW and Moynihan TJ (2011). Oncologic emergencies: pathophysiology, presentation, diagnosis, and treatment. *CA: A Cancer Journal for Clinicians*, 61(5): 287.

Loblaw DA et al. (2012). A 2011 updated systematic review and clinical practice guideline for the management of malignant extradural spinal cord compression. *International Journal of Radiation Oncology, Biology, Physics*, 84(2): 312–317.

Longo DL, Ropper AE and Ropper AH (2017). Acute spinal cord compression. *New England Journal of Medicine*, 376(14): 1358–1369.

Lyman GH, Lyman CH and Agboola O (2005). Risk models for predicting chemotherapy-induced neutropenia. *Oncologist*, 10(6): 427–437.

Minisola S et al. (2015). The diagnosis and management of hypercalcaemia. *BMJ*, 350(8011): h2723.

Mirrakhimov A (2015). Hypercalcemia of malignancy: an update on pathogenesis and management. (Review Article) (Report). *North American Journal of Medical Science*, 7(11): 483.

Mort D et al. (2008). *For better, for worse? A review of the care of patients who died within 30 days of receiving systemic anti-cancer therapy*. London: National Confidential Enquiry into Patient Outcome and Death.

Multinational Association of Supportive Care in Cancer (2019). *Identifying patients at Low Risk for FN Complications: Development and Validation of the MASCC Risk Index Score*. Available at: https://www.mascc.org/mascc-fn-risk-index-score.

National Chemotherapy Advisory Group (2009). *Chemotherapy Services in England: Ensuring Quality and Safety. A Report from the National Chemotherapy Advisory Group*. Available at: https://webarchive.nationalarchives.gov.uk/20130104232541/http://www.dh.gov.uk/prod_consum_dh/groups/dh_digitalassets/documents/digitalasset/dh_104501.pdf.

National Institute for Health and Care Excellence (2008). *Metastatic spinal cord compression in adults: risk assessment, diagnosis and management* (CG75). London: NICE.

National Institute for Health and Care Excellence (2012). *Neutropenic Sepsis: Prevention and Management of Neutropenic Sepsis in Cancer Patients* (CG151). London: NICE.

Parikh RB et al. (2013). Early specialty palliative care--translating data in oncology into practice. *New England Journal of Medicine*, 369(24): 2347–2351.

Prasad D and Schiff D (2005). Malignant spinal-cord compression. *The Lancet Oncology*, 6(1): 15–24.

Rachapalli V and Boucher LM (2014). Superior vena cava syndrome: role of the interventionalist. *Canadian Association of Radiologists Journal*, 65(2): 168–176.

Rhodes A et al. (2017). Surviving Sepsis Campaign: International Guidelines for Management of Sepsis and Septic Shock: 2016. *Intensive Care Medicine*, 43(3): 304–377.

Rowell NP and Gleeson FV (2002). Steroids, radiotherapy, chemotherapy and stents for superior vena caval obstruction in carcinoma of the bronchus: a systematic review. *Clinical Oncology*, 14(5): 338–351.

Savage P et al. (2014). Malignant spinal cord compression: NICE guidance, improvements and challenges. *QJM: monthly journal of the Association of Physicians*, 107(4): 277.

Schifferdecker B et al. (2005). Nonmalignant superior vena cava syndrome: pathophysiology and management. *Catheterization and Cardiovascular Interventions*, 65(3): 416–423.

Schrijvers D (2011). Emergencies in palliative care. *European Journal of Cancer*, 47: S359–S361.

Sculier JP et al. (1986). Superior vena caval obstruction syndrome in small cell lung cancer. *Cancer*, 57(4): 847–851.

Smith TJ et al. (2015). Recommendations for the use of WBC growth factors: American Society of Clinical Oncology Clinical Practice Guideline update. *Journal of Clinical Oncology: official journal of the American Society of Clinical Oncology*, 33(28): 3199.

Sternlicht H and Glezerman IG (2015). Hypercalcemia of malignancy and new treatment options. *Therapeutics and Clinical Risk Management*, 11: 1779.

Stewart, AF (2005). Clinical practice. Hypercalcemia associated with cancer. *The New England Journal of Medicine*, 352(4): 373.

Straka C et al. (2016). Review of evolving etiologies, implications and treatment strategies for the superior vena cava syndrome. *Springerplus*, 5: 229.

Talbot T et al. (2017). The burden of neutropenic sepsis in patients with advanced non-small cell lung cancer treated with single-agent docetaxel: a retrospective study. *Lung Cancer*, 113(C), 115–120.

Temel JS et al. (2010). Early palliative care for patients with metastatic non–small-cell lung cancer. *The New England Journal of Medicine*, 363(8): 733–742.

Ubogagu E and Harris DG (2012). Guideline for the management of terminal haemorrhage in palliative care patients with advanced cancer discharged home for end-of-life care. *BMJ Supportive and Palliative Care*, 2(4): 294–300.

van der Velden WJFM et al. (2014). Mucosal barrier injury, fever and infection in neutropenic patients with cancer: introducing the paradigm febrile mucositis. *British Journal of Haematology*, 167(4): 441–452.

Watson MS (2009). *Oxford Handbook of Palliative Care* (2nd ed.). Oxford: Oxford University Press.

Watson M et al. (2009). *Emergencies in Palliative Care* (2nd ed.). Oxford: Oxford University Press.

Warnock C (2016). Neutropenic sepsis: prevention, identification and treatment. *Nursing Standard*, 30(35): 51.

Welsh SJ and Strauss SJ (2012). Assessment of the patient with neutropenic sepsis. *British Journal of Hospital Medicine*, 73(6): C89.

White BD et al. (2008). Guidelines: Diagnosis and management of patients at risk of or with metastatic spinal cord compression: summary of NICE Guidance. *BMJ*, 337(7682): 1349–1351.

Wiese CHR et al. (2008). Treatment of palliative emergencies by paramedics. *The Middle European Journal of Medicine*, 120(17): 539–546.

Wiese CHR et al. (2013). International recommendations for outpatient palliative care and prehospital palliative emergencies – a prospective questionnaire-based investigation. *BMC Palliative Care*, 12(1): 10.

Wilson LD, Detterbeck FC and Yahalom J (2007). Superior vena cava syndrome with malignant causes. *The New England Journal of Medicine*, 356(18): 1862–1869.

Chapter 4

Symptom Management

Stephen Cox

Introduction

One of the highest priorities for patients with life-limiting illness is having the comfort of knowing that distressing symptoms can be managed day or night. In the past this would have been the role of general practice but the landscape has changed in the last decade or so and now the burden of symptom management, particularly at weekends and overnight, rests with the paramedic service. Symptom management in all specialties is based upon history taking, a thorough physical assessment, formulating the most likely cause and planning a treatment that is agreed with the patient and family. The challenge in palliative care is that time might be short and many treatments widely used elsewhere may be inappropriate for a patient with extensive life-limiting disease.

Patients are more than their disease and cannot be defined by it. They are people living in social and psychological frameworks, which are both *affected* by a life-limiting illness and have an *effect* on the severity of symptoms experienced. Treating a patient as a 'disease cluster' is totally at odds with whole person care. However, no matter how empathetic and understanding a paramedic is of a patient's situation, if they fail to treat symptoms then they fail the patient.

> *Tips for practice*
> *One method of experiencing palliative care is to work in a unit for a week or more either during a student rotation or after qualifying. Hospices will always welcome paramedic colleagues.*

This chapter looks at the most common symptoms experienced in palliative care. The evidence base in palliative care is still developing and a lot of the symptom management is derived from other specialties, therefore the management described in the chapter is a guide rather than a protocol and so local guidelines should also be referred to. Paramedics should always be aware of their own scope of practice when managing palliative emergencies and also abide their local NHS trust guidance.

Pain Management

Pain is a common symptom among patients receiving palliative care and often worsens as disease progresses. All too often, pain is poorly managed in both the community and secondary care (Smith and Saiki, 2015) and presents a clinician with a challenging task. Virtually all patients in the last year of life will experience pain at some stage and, in many, this pain is complex and difficult to manage.

Many patients with complex pain will be under the care of a hospice team alongside other specialist teams and the GP, all of whom are responsible for managing and monitoring symptoms. The aim of pain management is to maintain comfort to enable a patient to continue activities that they value. Good pain management supports both the patient and the wider family and reduces hospital admissions and out of hours calls. This section will focus on the nomenclature of pain and guidance on practical management.

Pain is expressed in many ways but has been defined by the International Association for the Study of Pain as:

> An unpleasant sensory and emotional experience associated with actual or potential tissue damage, or described in terms of such damage.
>
> (Treede et al., 2015)

This definition implies that pain is not just physical but also subjective and affects the psychological, functional and physical aspects of a patient's life. It is a complex subject. In essence, pain is what the patient says it is (McCaffery, 1994).

Pain is not a single entity; it is separated into a number of groups. In practice these groups often overlap, but to have a set of basic definitions is helpful when it comes to assessing pain. Watson et al. (2020) propose the following:

- **Acute pain** – characterised by its sudden onset. It typically responds well to analgesics and treating the underlying cause.

- **Chronic pain** – characterised by a gradual onset and persisting from weeks to months. It can be associated with behavioural, functional and personality changes and is frequently resistant to analgesics, even at high dose.

- **Nociceptive pain** – pain from an identified cause such as tumour or metastases. It is further divided into:

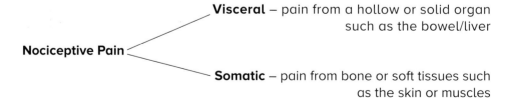

Nociceptive Pain

Visceral – pain from a hollow or solid organ such as the bowel/liver

Somatic – pain from bone or soft tissues such as the skin or muscles

- **Neuropathic pain** – derived from central or peripheral nerves. It typically follows a dermatome and has characteristic shooting, burning and tingling sensations. Neuropathic pain is further divided into three main groups depending on the source of the injury:

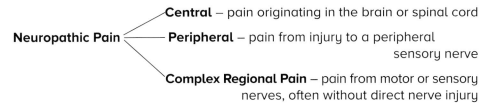

Neuropathic Pain

Central – pain originating in the brain or spinal cord

Peripheral – pain from injury to a peripheral sensory nerve

Complex Regional Pain – pain from motor or sensory nerves, often without direct nerve injury

Pain can also be referred from the organ affected via the nervous system to other parts of the body. For example, pain from a prolapsed lumbar disc may be felt in the leg via the sciatic nerve. Pain from a pancreatic tumour is often first felt in the lower thoracic spine referred via the coeliac plexus.

Patterns of pain are descriptions of the temporal (physical) aspects of pain:

- Background pain is a persistent pain or a pain lasting for many hours. This pattern of pain is best treated by a long acting analgesic.

- Breakthrough pain is an exacerbation of pain, usually spontaneous, which occurs despite relatively stable background pain.

- Incident pain is pain on activity such as movement, during nursing care or during a dressing change.

- Total pain is an important topic in end of life and palliative care. It describes pain that is not only physical but is also driven by psychological, social and spiritual needs. Total pain needs a total approach; unless all elements of this pain are addressed then it persists and usually requires the involvement of a specialist multidisciplinary team.

(Mehta and Chan, 2008)

Pain Assessment

Uncontrolled or poorly controlled pain is a source of great distress to both patients and families. A paramedic team meeting a patient for the first time has a critical role in managing a complex situation.

An accurate assessment of pain is essential before planning any treatment. The most frequently used assessments are the 'verbal rating scale' (no pain to worst pain imaginable), the '0–10 numeric scale', 'visual analogue scale' and the 'faces scale' (☺ to ☹). This will not suffice for assessing pain in patients needing a palliative approach. Pain in this group is more complex. It can be approached by using two assessments that complement each other. Many trusts have their own pain assessment protocols.

Thomas and Monaghan (2014) suggest an 'alphabet approach' first:

- O – **Onset** – When did this pain start?
  - Acute or chronic pain, or acute on chronic?
- P – **Provoke** – What made the pain come on? Was it at rest or during activity?
  - Background pain or incident pain?
- Q – **Quality** – What is the character of the pain? Sharp, dull, heavy, burning, stinging etc?
  - Somatic, visceral, neuropathic or a mix of pain?
- R – **Region** – Where is the pain occurring and is it spreading elsewhere?
  - Is this referred pain?
- S – **Severity and symptoms** – Is the patient crying with pain or sitting quietly?
  - Assess with a simple 1–10 pain scale.

The second task is to carry out an assessment of the physical, social and psychological issues that may be causing or worsening the pain.

- **Physical** – Are these symptoms related to the *underlying disease*, e.g. cancer, bowel obstruction, pleural effusion etc?
  - Are they related to *treatments* for the disease, e.g. chemotherapy, radiotherapy or drug side effects?
  - Consider other *background conditions* such as cardiac or musculoskeletal disease.
- **Sociological** – Illness is not just a physical experience. It is expressed through sociological structures and these structures can aid or harm the patient. A close and supportive family may help a patient make some sense of the situation they are in, appreciate the life they have led, come to terms with regret. Destructive relationships can lead to anger, blame and regret. Seeing the patient in their social context yet acknowledging them as an individual is central to a deeper and more therapeutic relationship with a patient. Knowing what gives the patient meaning and purpose in their lives, what energises them or gives pleasure, builds trust and a therapeutic relationship.
- **Psychological** – Psychological factors have a profound influence on how patients experience and express pain. Behavioural and emotional responses to pain are underpinned by psychological issues. Fear, depression, anxiety and pain affect all other issues and pain cannot be fully assessed unless the psychological aspects are addressed. Asking how the patient's mood has been (depression?), what is troubling them most (anxiety, fear?), or how they see the future can be a pathway into psychological issues.
- **Total pain** – Discussing psychological and sociological aspects of pain are central in understanding and helping a patient with total pain. Total pain

was first described by Cecily Saunders (the founder of the modern hospice movement) in the *Prescribers Journal* (Saunders, 1964). She was struck by a comment from a patient who said, 'all of me is wrong'. Behind this comment was a raft of psychological and social issues driving their pain. Total pain contrasts starkly to acute pain – the latter has meaning and leads to investigations and treatment; total pain on the other hand 'is meaningless' (Saunders, 1970). Many patients have this multi-layered complex of symptoms, which worsen pain and are not resolved by opioids. Two characteristics of patients with total pain are, first, that 'nothing works' (whether that be drugs or the problems with transport and appointments) and second, that they are often patients on rapidly escalating analgesics with no benefit. Multidisciplinary teams in hospices can help explore in depth the underlying factors in total pain.

Pain Assessment in Patients with Cognitive Impairment

Assessing pain in a patient with cognitive impairment can be a challenge. The aim is to get a clear description of the pain, identify the causes if possible, and make a plan with the family and carers. The *Scottish Palliative Care Guidelines* (NHS Scotland, 2019) provide a comprehensive approach; below is a brief summary.

The first duty is to identify whether the patient has capacity to make decisions about pain and can describe it.

1. Perform the two-stage capacity screen (SCIE, 2019).
2. If no capacity, check for power of attorney or written instructions.
3. If neither are present, treat in 'best interests' but with the involvement and agreement of as many family members and carers as possible.

Use the family and carers' observations:

- How is pain normally expressed?
- Check for patient-held notes.
- Are there any other medical problems causing pain?

Enhance communications:

- Check the need for hearing aids and glasses.
- Use simple language.
- Repeat questions to the patient and check the patient understands.

Observe:

- facial expressions
- body movements
- attempts to verbalise.

Is pain the problem?

- Fear and anxiety worsen pain.
- Is delirium present?
- Is there another issue such as constipation, pressure sores or urine infection?

Two validated screening tools are available. The DISDAT tool (2006) is an assessment completed by family or carers that helps set a baseline for the patient. The PAINAD tool is shown below (Table 4.1) and is quick to complete (Jordan, 2011).

Table 4.1 Pain Assessment in Advanced Dementia (PAINAD) scale

Items	0	1	2	Score
Breathing independent of vocalisation	Normal	Occasional laboured breathing. Short period of hyperventilation.	Noisy laboured breathing. Long period of hyperventilation. Cheyne-Stokes respirations.	
Negative vocalisation	None	Occasional moan or groan. Low-level speech with a negative or disapproving quality.	Repeated troubled calling out. Loud moaning or groaning. Crying.	
Facial expression	Smiling or inexpressive	Sad. Frightened. Frown.	Facial grimacing.	
Body language	Relaxed	Tense. Distressed pacing. Fidgeting.	Rigid. Fists clenched. Knees pulled up. Pulling or pushing away. Striking out.	
Consolability	No need to console	Distracted or reassured by voice or touch.	Unable to console, distract or reassure.	
Total score indicates degree of pain: 0 = none; 10 = severe				

(Jordan, 2011)

The World Health Organization (WHO) Pain Ladder

The WHO three-step ladder is the most widely accepted guideline for managing pain (Figure 4.1). It was designed for cancer-related pain and not chronic pain from other causes. In practice, Step 2 is often omitted if strong opioids are readily available. The WHO chart was designed for use across the world but in many areas strong opioids are not easily obtained. Morphine remains the gold standard opioid, but contact the hospice or GP if the pain is inadequately controlled.

The pain ladder has been criticised for not including newer treatments and interventions such as nerve blocks, methadone and ketamine. These interventions are approved by WHO but do not appear on the pain ladder (Carlson, 2016). Leave a pain chart for the patient to use; this will help the next professional the patient sees.

Opioids for Pain

All opioids are effective drugs for the relief of pain in advanced life-threatening disease. Despite many fears and misunderstandings, opioids are very safe if used carefully. Addiction and misuse of opioids tends to occur most frequently when used for chronic non-malignant pain and is very uncommon in patients nearing the end of life (Twycross and Wilcock, 2018).

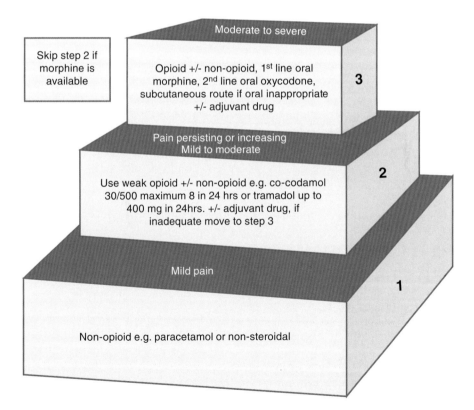

Figure 4.1   WHO Pain Ladder

Source: Adapted with the kind permission of the World Health Organization from 'WHO's cancer pain ladder for adults' (2019)

In hospice practice, drugs are usually administered subcutaneously (SC) rather than intramuscularly (IM) or intravenously (IV). The speed of action of the SC route is a little slower than IV but much more comfortable for the patient. Many patients have extensive oedema or are difficult to cannulate and SC injections via a plastic port in the skin are painless.

Start cautiously, use low doses initially – start at the lowest dose on the community prescription chart unless a higher dose has been used in the preceding days. Use the end of life care prescribing guidelines used by your Trust or the local hospice guidelines. The guidelines will cover the circumstances in which opioids can be given, doses and what to prescribe if end of life medications and prescribing chart are in the house.

Naloxone and Opioid-Induced Respiratory Depression

Naloxone is an opioid receptor antagonist and is remarkably safe if used carefully. It is ineffective if given orally but works rapidly if given IV (1–2 minutes). IM and SC doses act within 2–5 minutes. Patients who are opioid toxic can look as though they are dying, and it is important that opioid overdose is detected and the situation reversed. The key signs are drowsiness or unconsciousness *with a respiratory rate of 8 per minute or less*. Pinpoint pupils are not a reliable sign and should be ignored (Twycross and Wilcock, 2018).

If the patient has a respiratory rate around 8 but is easily rousable and not cyanosed then omit the next dose of opioid and observe closely.

Opioid antagonism by naloxone lasts 15–75 minutes. If the patient is taking modified-release opioids these can be active for 12–24 hours, instant relief opioids for around 4 hours (BNF, 2019). Patients may therefore need multiple doses or a continuous infusion.

Reversing Opioid Overdoses

Overdoses rarely occur due to the patient deliberately taking excessive drugs. More commonly opioids accumulate due to reduced renal clearance or as a result of opioid rotation particularly if long-acting drugs are involved.

Reversing overdose is a specialist treatment and is best done under the guidance of hospice clinicians or in the emergency department. However, in an emergency there is no harm in starting naloxone until advice is available.

To reverse respiratory depression (JRCALC, 2019):

1. Stop the opioid.

2. Administer naloxone slowly in three-minute intervals at a concentration of 400 micrograms in 1 ml ampoule IV. The aim is for slow administration of the drug to avoid a surge of pain from complete antagonism of opoid. If the IV/IO route is unavailable then administer 400 micrograms IM.

3. Titrate the dose against respiratory rate NOT level of consciousness; give dose every 2 minutes until respiratory rate is restored.

4. Consider oxygen if saturations are 94% or less.

Naloxone is not effective in buprenorphine overdose. In this case, seek help from the emergency department.

Understand the Relative Strengths of Opioids

The relative strengths of opioids are more of an art than a science and experts disagree. Become familiar with the agreed conversion charts in your locality or check the current conversions in a trusted source, such as the Palliative Care Network Guidlines Plus (see further reading section for more information).

The Leeds Opioid Conversion Guide (Leeds Community Healthcare and St Gemma's Hospice, 2016) is an example of the conversion charts available (Figure 4.2).

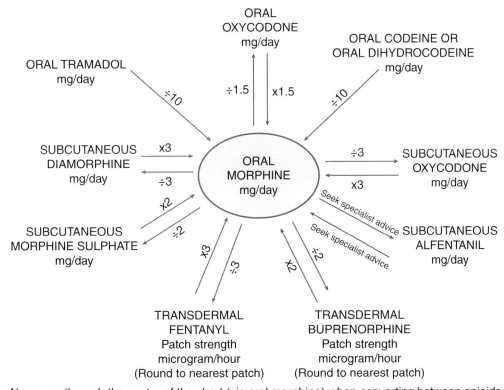

Always go through the centre of the chart (via oral morphine) when converting between opioids

> **NOTE:** All calculations and rationale must be documented in the patient's record, including those for prn doses.
>
> Clinical judgment should be applied, considering: underlying clinical situation; comorbidity (e.g. renal or liver impairment); drug interactions; nature of pain and its opioid responsiveness; other pain interventions; symptoms being managed by opioid; toxicity of current opioid previous opioid doses and adherence; rapidity of opioid escalation; use of larger doses; switches involving change of route; malabsorption issues; reason for switching. These factors **may** necessitate an empirical reduction in dose of the replacement opioid re-titration.
>
> For further advice contact your Local Specialist Palliative Care Service.

Figure 4.2   The Leeds Opioid Conversion Guide for Adult Palliative Care Patients
Source: Reproduced with the kind permission of the Leeds Palliative Care Network

Any calculations and the rationale for them should be recorded in the patient notes. This chart is no more than a guide; clinical conditions such as renal or hepatic failure will affect drug sensitivity. Many centres advise a reduction in the dose of an opioid of up to 50% when switching drugs, for example from morphine to oxycodone.

Understand the Side Effects

Opioid side effects are common and include nausea, vomiting, drowsiness, fatigue and constipation. If opioid levels become toxic then the patient may complain of hallucinations, tremors, drowsiness and a heightened sensitivity to pain (hyperalgesia) (Twycross and Wilcock, 2018). Opioids suppress the respiratory centre, but this effect is antagonised by pain, so if used appropriately, there is very little risk of this occurring.

Use Cautiously in Renal Impairment

The renal function of a patient may not be available, though some community charts include the most recent estimated glomerular filtration rate (eGFR) on the front cover. As a rule morphine (which is renally excreted) is avoided if the GFR is 30 or less. Some clinicians will use oxycodone in this situation. Oxycodone though is also renally excreted, but the side effects are better tolerated. If renal failure is present, seek specialist advice; alternatives such as alfentanil in a continuous infusion and patches may be more appropriate. The Renal Drug Handbook provides guidance on appropriate doses (Ashley and Currie, 2019) as does the BNF (2019).

Commonly Used Drugs

Non-Opioid Analgesics

Paracetamol – Paracetamol is a synthetic non-opioid analgesic and anti-pyretic. Paracetamol acts on the anti-inflammatory pathway, inhibits other pain pathways and interacts with the opioid systems to enhance the analgesic effect. However, there is little evidence to support or refute the use of paracetamol alongside opioids.

Non-Steroidal Anti-Inflammatory Drugs (NSAIDs)

This group of drugs reduce inflammation-induced pain. The evidence base in palliative care is poor for NSAIDs; however, they are widely used on a case-by-case basis as an adjuvant drug in all types of pain, particularly bone metastases. They have the added benefit of treating cancer-induced pyrexia.

Inflammation from tumours releases prostaglandins that stimulate pain in peripheral nerves and also trigger a response in the brain that further stimulates pain. NSAIDs interfere with both of these pathways (Twycross and Wilcock, 2019).

Most NSAIDs have numerous side effects, most notably peptic and small bowel ulceration, and deranged clotting and platelet function. They should be used with caution in patients with cardiovascular disease (Wood et al., 2018).

Weak Opioids

Codeine – Codeine is a weak opioid about a tenth the strength of morphine. A small percentage is converted to morphine, but response is very varied. Some individuals produce an enzyme that can block codeine and hence get little benefit. It is often combined with paracetamol though the benefit of this is unproven, and Step 2 of the WHO pathway can be omitted if morphine is available.

Tramadol – There is very little role for a weak opioid like tramadol (or codeine) if morphine is available. Tramadol is a weak synthetic opioid around a tenth of the strength of morphine. It is derived from codeine, safe in renal failure but compared to morphine it acts relatively slowly (Leppert and Luczak, 2005).

Serotonin syndrome – If tramadol is taken with a second drug, both of which interfere with pre-synaptic serotonin reuptake (tramadol and many antidepressants, for example), then serotonin syndrome can occur. This is a rare event but consider it if the patient is delirious or has a high temperature (Buckley et al., 2014)

Strong Opioids

Morphine – Morphine is the active constituent of opium and it works via specific opioid receptors peripherally and in the central nervous system. In cancer and inflammatory pain, the number of receptors increases and endogenous opioids are released. In bone and neuropathic pain, the opposite happens and receptors decrease, which probably explains the relatively poor effectiveness of opioids in these conditions. NICE recommend morphine as the first-line drug when opioids are indicated (NICE, 2012).

Oxycodone – This opiate is very similar to morphine but probably works on a wider range of receptors. It is approximately twice as potent as morphine and is a semi-synthetic compound. The active metabolites are excreted in both the liver and kidneys, and oxycodone should be avoided in moderate to severe liver failure. Oxycodone can be used cautiously in renal impairment, but once the eGFR falls below 30, alternatives should be considered (Ashley and Currie, 2019).

Analgesic Patches

There are three drugs in palliative care delivered by the transdermal route: buprenorphine, fentanyl and lidocaine. Buprenorphine and fentanyl work on the same receptors as morphine. Both are potent analgesics. Patches are not started as a first-line treatment or in patients who are 'opioid naïve'. Patches are indicated when an effective oral or subcutaneous dose is established: the dose can then be converted to a patch dose.

Patches are useful when swallowing, patient compliance or poor gut absorption is an issue (NICE, 2012). They are not for use with unstable or acute pain as it can take between 3 and 36 hours for them to become effective. Patch doses are less constipating than oral drugs.

Lidocaine patches contain a local anaesthetic in a slow-release formulation. They can be used for neuropathic pain, though there is minimal evidence to support their use (Finnerup et al., 2015).

Be careful with patches: the lowest patch strength of buprenorphine (5 microgram/h) is suitable for opioid-naïve patients, and the equivalent oral morphine dose is

12 mg/24 hrs. The lowest patch strength of fentanyl (12 microgram/h) is equivalent to 43 mg oral morphine and should not be used in opioid-naïve patients (Dickman, 2012).

Alfentanil – Alfentanil is a synthetic opioid in the same class of drug as fentanyl. It is most commonly used as a continuous subcutaneous infusion (CSCI) on specialist advice. It is a useful alternative to morphine and oxycodone in the presence of renal failure. The valuable feature of alfentanil is its speed of action; single doses are effective within a minute and the analgesic effect can last for up to thirty minutes. With such a short duration of action alfentanil is mainly used as a CSCI or as an SC injection for incident pain such as painful dressing changes (Twycross and Wilcock, 2019).

Fentanyl – In palliative care fentanyl is widely used as a transdermal patch. It is very similar to morphine in that it is a powerful mu-opioid receptor agonist. It is safe to use in patients with end-stage renal failure. Fentanyl is also produced as an IM or SC injection. It is rarely used on palliative care units but more commonly used for post-operative pain.

Transmucosal fentanyl is helpful in treating incident pain as serum levels peak after a few minutes and the effect lasts for around thirty minutes. This method needs good patient cooperation to titrate the dose. These formulations are expensive.

Adjuvant Drugs

Adjuvant drugs are a group of analgesics that support or complement opioids. Adjuvants have an important role particularly when the pain has a 'mixed' picture or in circumstances where opioids are relatively ineffective, such as in neuropathic pain. It could be argued that all pain is 'mixed', i.e. contains both nociceptive and neuropathic elements and adjuvants are widely used on that assumption. Adjuvant drugs include the following:

- amitriptyline (and other antidepressants) for neuropathic pain
- bisphosphonates for bone pain
- pregabalin or gabapentin for neuropathic and bone pain
- ketamine or methadone for intractable complex pain – these work on a set of receptors that are not accessible to opioids. They are only used under specialist guidance.

Amitriptyline or gabapentin are the first-line drugs when treating neuropathic pain. Second-line drugs include imipramine and duloxetine. These drugs work in the dorsal horn to subdue ectopic nerve activity. Neuropathic pain is sometimes sensitive to opioids (Finnerup, 2015).

Tapentadol

This drug is relatively new and an alternative drug to strong opioids. It is a relatively weak opioid receptor agonist but is a relatively powerful noradrenaline reuptake inhibitor similar to duloxetine. Despite its weak opioid effect tapentadol probably works via the synergistic effect of its pharmacological actions. It is an alternative to strong opioids, particularly if opioid side effects are an issue (Wood et al., 2018)

Pain Pathways and Sites of Action

Specific Pain Presentations

Metastatic bone pain is usually a deep aching sensation over a localised point. Bone pain is often opioid sensitive but frequently needs adjuvant drugs, especially paracetamol and NSAIDs. If pain persists then radiotherapy and IV bisphosphonates are indicated.

Headaches from raised intracranial pressure may occur with primary or secondary cerebral tumours. Patients may complain of headaches or head pressure on lying flat or on waking. Analgesics are usually ineffective; the most effective treatment is high dose dexamethasone (8 mg twice a day) together with an urgent referral to oncology for assessment (Watson et al., 2020).

Liver capsule pain is associated with a deep pain in the right upper quadrant, often worse on coughing or deep inspiration. The liver will usually feel enlarged and contain metastatic deposits. Dexamethasone is the drug of choice; liver capsule pain is often insensitive to opioids. See Figure 4.3 which illustrates the pain pathways and the relevant medications.

Non-Pharmacological Approaches

At the end of life, patients may derive more comfort and support from the care the paramedic gives than any drug. Attention to the small details matters. Are they comfortable? Can they reach the phone? What is really troubling them, is it pain or distress or fear?

It matters that clinicians are warm, friendly and view the whole person and not just the symptom. The clinician is often the drug. Kindness, thoughtfulness and a listening ear can be more potent than opioids.

Key Points

- Good analgesic control of pain is a right, especially at end of life.
- Be familiar with all the opiates and side effects.
- Acute pain must be viewed as an emergency and treated appropriately.
- Morphine is a safe drug when used carefully; if possible check a recent renal function.
- If reversing opioid-induced respiratory suppression, treat the respiratory rate and not the level of consciousness.
- Gabapentin, pregabalin, amitriptyline or duloxetine should be considered for patients with neuropathic cancer pain that is only partially responsive to opioid analgesia.
- If necessary, call the hospice teams; they are there to help.

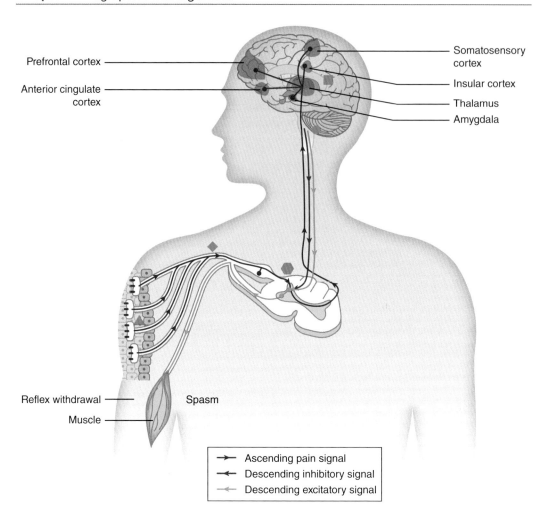

Sites of Action		Medications
▲	Peripherally (at the nociceptor cells)	NSAIDs, opioids, tramadol
◆	Peripherally (along the nociceptor nerve)	Local anaesthetics, anticonvulsants
■	Centrally, various brain sites	Paracetamol, anticonvulsants, opioids, tramadol
●	Descending inhibitory pathway in spinal cord	Opioids, tramadol, tricyclic antidepressants, SNRIs such as duloxetine
⬡	Dorsal horn of spinal cord	Anticonvulsants, e.g. gabapentin and pregabalin, opioids, tramadol, tricyclic antidepressants, SNRIs

Figure 4.3   Pain pathways and sites of action

Nausea and Vomiting

Nausea and vomiting are common symptoms in palliative care. Around 50% of patients with advanced malignancy or end-stage heart failure are affected; around 30% of patients with renal failure are affected.

- **Nausea** occurs most frequently in haematological cancers and renal failure.
- **Vomiting** is most common in gastrointestinal, gynaecological and breast cancers.

As cancers and organ failure progress, so does the incidence of nausea and vomiting. In the last weeks of life these distressing symptoms affects up to 75% of patients dying from all causes (Harris, 2010). They are distinct symptoms, which may occur together or entirely separately.

- **Nausea** is a feeling of needing to vomit. It is unpleasant and often accompanied by sweating, fast pulse rate and excess saliva.
- **Vomiting** is the actual expulsion of stomach and small bowel contents through the mouth. This is usually forceful, and the vomit projected.

> The word 'vomit' derives from the Latin 'vomitorium'. Many sources describe the vomitorium as a place where Romans went to vomit in order to keep eating – this is probably myth. It is more likely that the word derives from the name given to the exits at the Colosseum, which were narrow passages where people flowed out of the stadium. The word 'spew' comes from a Latin word to spit, but was adapted in Old English to include vomiting and later to describe the dispersing of vomit. Watching a crowd leave a stadium perfectly illustrates this: the crowd leave via a narrow passage (a vomitorium), then disperse outside the ground (spew).

The memory of vomiting lasts long in the mind; for a patient with advanced disease, the feeling of being on the verge of vomiting or vomiting many times a day is extremely distressing.

Mechanisms of Vomiting

Vomiting is a complex mechanism. If the vomiting centre is triggered, a number of events occur within a fraction of a second (Figure 4.4):

- **Breathing is halted** to stop the inhalation of vomit.
- **Peristalsis is reversed** and the stomach fills with fluid from the small intestine.
- **The diaphragm contracts** and abdominal muscles tighten to force the vomit out.

- **The lower oesophageal sphincter (LES) relaxes** and allows direct access to the mouth.

- **The soft palate closes the glottis** to stop fluid pouring into the lungs.

Nausea and vomiting in palliative patients is often complex and involves a number of causes. For many patients, nausea is far more debilitating than occasional vomiting, whereas persistent vomiting is both physically, socially and psychologically debilitating.

However, for palliative patients vomiting is a feared symptom, and many patients rate vomiting more troublesome than pain.

The Emetic Pathway – What Initiates Vomiting?

A number of structures feed signals to the vomiting centre in the brain. Two brainstem areas, the chemotactic trigger zone (CTZ) and the vomiting centre, are areas that are often taught as separate structures but are in fact interconnected by complex neural networks.

The **CTZ** is activated by chemicals in the blood and cerebrospinal fluid and by signals from the vagus and vestibular nerves. The receptors in this area, mostly dopamine, are triggered by a range of chemicals including calcium, but most crucially by opioid drugs.

The **cerebral cortex** is thought to be stimulated via histamine and acetylcholine receptors, which are triggered by anxiety, fear, raised intracranial pressure and irritation of the meninges lining the brain.

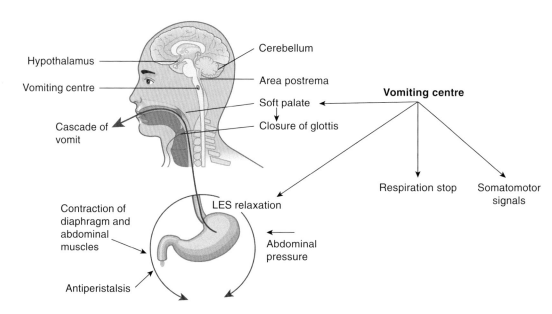

Figure 4.4 Act of vomiting

The **vestibular nuclei** are triggered by movement via the balance mechanism of the middle ear. This is mediated by histamine.

The **gastrointestinal (GI) tract** directly stimulates the vomiting centre via the release of serotonin (5-HT). Serotonin is released in response to radiotherapy, bacterial exotoxins and a wide range of drugs. A second group of neurotransmitters (histamine and acetylcholine) are stimulated by bowel distortion, such as tumour growth and bowel obstruction. This is transmitted to the brain via the vagus nerve.

The GI tract is often termed 'the gut brain'; the complexity of neurotransmitters it releases and their impact on the 'head brain' are poorly understood at present.

Nausea and Vomiting – Clinical Triggers

It is critically important to **view nausea and vomiting as a symptom not a disease**. They always have a cause; the job of the paramedic is, as far as possible, to identify the cause in order to determine the best treatment.

An effective approach is to work through the body methodically from head to anus. The basis of all diagnoses is an accurate history and examination, and nausea and vomiting are usually rich in history, signs and symptoms. Thomas and Monaghan (2014) provide an excellent source of information on examination techniques.

Examine the patient thoroughly – check the fundi, listen to the chest, examine the abdomen, percuss for fluid or air, and palpate the abdominal structures.

Each of the causes in Figure 4.5 have a distinct presenting sign or symptom. In palliative care there is often more than one cause of nausea and vomiting. However, by breaking the problem down into symptoms, the complexity of the presenting situation can be worked through.

Key Features

Presenting Sign or Symptom

Feeling of fullness after small volumes of food or fluid, hiccups, reflux?

Likely causes are impaired gastric emptying or duodenal obstruction.

Think

- **Drugs** – particularly opioids and anticholinergics such as hyoscine.
- **Ascites** – examine for shifting dullness in a distended abdomen.
- **Hepatomegaly** – a large liver is usually easy to palpate.
- **Tumour** – compressing the duodenum or stomach.

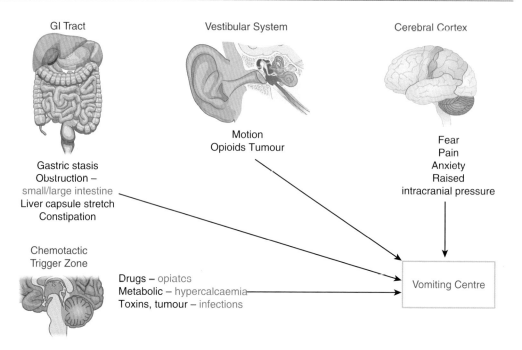

GI Tract

Vestibular System

Cerebral Cortex

Motion
Opioids Tumour

Fear
Pain
Anxiety
Raised
intracranial pressure

Gastric stasis
Obstruction –
small/large intestine
Liver capsule stretch
Constipation

Chemotactic
Trigger Zone

Drugs – opiates
Metabolic – hypercalcaemia
Toxins, tumour – infections

Vomiting Centre

Figure 4.5   Causes of vomiting and nausea

Presenting Sign or Symptom

Vomiting and the patient has delirium?

Think

- **Drugs** – opioids, digoxin toxicity, antifungals (ketoconazole), SSRIs (e.g., paroxetine).
- **Chemotherapy** – hypomagnesemia after chemotherapy can cause delirium and vomiting.
- **Metabolic causes** – renal and hepatic failure can alter sodium or calcium.
- **Toxins** – from ischaemic bowel, bowel obstruction, tumour toxins and infection.

Presenting Sign or Symptom

Vomiting undigested food or bile associated with abdominal pain?

Think

- **Visceral and serosal causes** – bowel obstruction, faecal impaction, liver capsule stretch and prolonged coughing.

Presenting Sign or Symptom

Vomiting associated with headache?

Think

- **Raised intracranial pressure** – the associated headache is often worse on waking.
- **Meningeal infiltration** – presents with personality changes, visual hallucinations, mood changes and delirium.

Presenting Sign or Symptom

Vomiting associated with movement?

Think

- **Vestibular** causes such as motion sickness and opioid drugs. Has the patient just had an ambulance journey?

Presenting Sign or Symptom

Vomiting associated with anxiety?

Think

- **Cortical** vomiting can often be triggered by memories, smells and learned behaviour. The amygdala is a complex area of the brain that stores previous memories and stimuli. When triggered, for example by a smell, a shower of neurotransmitters is released. Interestingly, patients with a damaged amygdala lose all fear of learned threats such as snakes.

Assessment and Examination

All patients should be assessed for the following:

- Dehydration
- Sepsis
- Delirium.

The abdomen should also be examined. To examine the abdomen do the following:

- Listen for bowel obstruction (scanty or absent bowel sounds).
- Palpate – is the liver or spleen enlarged?
- Look for ascites and constipation.
- Check for a succussion splash – listen over the stomach with a stethoscope and gently rock the patient. Splashing sounds indicate gastric stasis or outflow obstruction.

Ask all patients about any anxieties and concerns they have concerning their symptoms or about their diagnosis and disease progression in general.

Management of Nausea and Vomiting

Deciding which drug to use will be based upon a combination of clinical examination and a 'best guess' at the cause. Local hospices or trusts may have their own treatment regime. Table 4.2 is a suggested protocol arranged by likely cause. Table 4.3 details commonly used drugs for managing symptoms of nausea and vomiting.

Table 4.2 Suggested protocol for managing nausea and vomiting

Cause	First Line	Second Line
Gastric stasis	Metoclopramide O/SC/CSCI	Domperidone O
Abdominal causes (e.g. bowel obstruction)	Levomepromazine SC/CSCI	Cyclizine SC/CSCI
Cranial	Cyclizine SC/CSCI	Haloperidol O/SC
Chemical	Haloperidol O/SC/CSCI	Levomepromazine SC/ CSCI or ondansetron/ granisetron
Cortical	Levomepromazine O/SC/CSCI	Oxazepam/lorazepam SL
Vestibular	Levomepromazine O/SC/CSCI	Cyclizine O/SC/CSCI (use water as diluent)

O = oral; SC = subcutaneous; SL = sublingual; CSCI = continuous subcutaneous infusion.
Obtain current dosing regimens from Palliative Care Adult Network Guidelines or BNF.

(Adapted Stephenson and Davies, 2006; Twycross and Wilcock, 2018)

Table 4.3 Commonly used drugs

Drug Action	Clinical Use	Side Effects	Comments
Metoclopramide Prokinetic – empties the stomach and encourages bowel peristalsis	Impaired gastric emptying, partial bowel obstruction	Colic Extrapyramidal side effects, tardive dyskinesia. Check current BNF for advice. Affects QT interval.* Avoid in Parkinson's disease.	Do not use in complete bowel obstruction, perforation or gut bleeding. Avoid in renal failure.
Domperidone Prokinetic	Impaired gastric emptying	Colic Safe in Parkinson's disease. Affects QTc interval.*	Can be given rectally.
Cyclizine Acts in the brain	There is no good palliative care evidence for using cyclizine.	Sedating even at low doses, dry mouth, constipation.	Avoid in cardiac failure. Sometimes used if brain metastases are present. Does not affect seizure threshold.
Levomepromazine Has broad spectrum effect, acts in all sites, useful in all causes of nausea and vomiting	First line drug if cause of nausea and vomiting is uncertain.	Extrapyramidal side effects. Sedating at higher doses. Theoretically reduces seizure threshold,** caution when brain metastases present. Affects QTc interval.*	Widely used as a first-line drug. Avoid in Parkinson's disease.
Haloperidol Acts in the brain	First line in nausea and vomiting from chemical causes, particularly if delirium present.	Extrapyramidal side effects. Affects QT interval.* Theoretically reduces seizure threshold.**	Avoid in Parkinson's disease.

(continued)

Table 4.3 Commonly used drugs (*continued*)

Drug Action	Clinical Use	Side Effects	Comments
Olanzapine Acts in the brain	First-line drug if cause of nausea and vomiting is uncertain.	Theoretically reduces seizure threshold.** Sedating at higher doses.	Useful in delirium.
Ondansetron **Granisetron** Has broad spectrum effect	First-/second-line in chemical causes, bowel obstruction and renal failure.	Constipation Headache Affects QT interval.*	Used widely for chemotherapy induced nausea/ vomiting.

*A small number of the population show a prolonged QT interval on ECG. This is usually genetic. A prolonged QT interval can give rise to a life-threatening arrhythmia when certain drugs are used. The relevance in palliative care depends to some extent on prognosis. All drugs that prolong the QT interval are clearly marked in the BNF.

**A seizure threshold is the balance between stimulatory and inhibitory activity in the brain. Some drugs upset this balance putting the patient at risk of fits.

(Adapted from Stephenson and Davies, 2006; Twycross and Wilcock, 2018)

Key Points

- Nausea and vomiting are common, particularly in the last few weeks of life.

- It is distressing for both patient and carers.

- Look carefully for a cause – this will guide management.

- Seek further advice from the palliative care team if bowel obstruction or cerebral metastases are suspected.

Breathlessness

Breathlessness is an important and very common symptom in advanced disease. Breathlessness causes considerable distress and disability, and is a complex symptom to manage. Best practice invokes a range of pharmacological and non-pharmacological interventions involving a 'whole team' approach.

Breathlessness is a *subjective* experience of breathing discomfort. This experience consists of *qualitatively* distinct sensations such as chest tightness, air hunger or effort in breathing. Breathlessness derives from a mix of social, physiological and psychological factors and the key point is that the experience of breathlessness is generated in the brain and only the patient can fully experience its impact. Breathlessness is not a symptom that can be understood by undertaking physiological investigations in isolation (Booth et al., 2015).

The prevalence of breathlessness is high; it affects around 80% of patients with lung cancer, 90% in congestive cardiac failure and 95% of patients with chronic obstructive pulmonary disease (COPD) (Currow et al., 2010).

Assessment

The Medical Research Council's dyspnoea scale for grading the degree of a patient's breathlessness is widely used by paramedics and inpatient units:

1. Not troubled by breathlessness except on strenuous exercise.

2. Short of breath when hurrying or walking up a slight hill.

3. Walks slower than contemporaries on the level because of breathlessness, or has to stop for breath when walking at own pace.

4. Stops for breath after about 100 m or after a few minutes on the level.

5. Too breathless to leave the house, or breathless when dressing or undressing.

(MRC, 2008)

This scale does not measure breathlessness itself but perceived respiratory disability. Other scales have been proposed but none have been widely adopted for general use.

Chronic breathlessness has been promoted as a distinct clinical syndrome and is defined as:

> ... breathlessness that persists despite optimal treatment of the underlying pathophysiology and results in disability.

(Johnson and Yorke, 2017)

This syndrome is composed of three events that lead to a cycle of distressing breathlessness: inefficient breathing, anxiety and muscle deterioration. There are interventions to help but as in all situations, the priority is to first treat the treatable and reverse the reversible.

Reversible Causes

The definition above stresses the importance of recognising the underlying reversible causes of breathlessness. Paramedic training emphasises that breathlessness is often derived from other systems apart from the lungs. The list of causes is long, but the most common are:

- **Respiratory:**
  - pneumonia
  - lung cancer
  - COPD

- interstitial disease (e.g. pulmonary fibrosis)

- pleural effusion

- pulmonary embolus.

- **Cardiac:**

  - pericardial effusion

  - congestive cardiac failure

  - arrhythmias.

- **Systemic:**

  - anaemia

  - sepsis

  - renal failure.

- **Psychological:**

  - anxiety/panic episodes

  - depression.

The 'Breathing, Thinking, Functioning' Model

The Cambridge Breathless Intervention Service have developed a model to aid self-management of long-term breathlessness (Figure 4.6). The model highlights the three essential elements that drive the sensation of breathlessness and stresses the interconnection between them (Spathis et al., 2017).

- **Breathing domain** – Patients with advanced lung disease are likely to develop dysfunctional breathing patterns. This is driven by the need to 'get more air' and subconsciously alter their breathing rate and use the upper muscles of the chest to breathe rather than the diaphragm. These muscles are liable to fatigue (unlike the diaphragm) and therefore increase the intensity of breathlessness.

- **Thinking domain** – If a patient has dysfunctional breathing this can generate a fear of being breathless, which then increases the sensation of breathlessness. This vicious cycle, if left unchecked, triggers panic and the frequent involvement of paramedics. This is probably mediated in the cortico-limbic area of the brain where breathing and emotion perception are both sited.

- **Functioning domain** – A further vicious cycle now develops. As breathlessness is an unpleasant experience, the natural reaction is to become less active. Inactivity leads to muscle fibre atrophy, and the less fit the patient is, the more the breathlessness deteriorates.

Breathlessness is not reliably predicted by the severity of the lung pathology; unhelpful emotions and behaviours exacerbate and maintain the recurrence of the symptom.

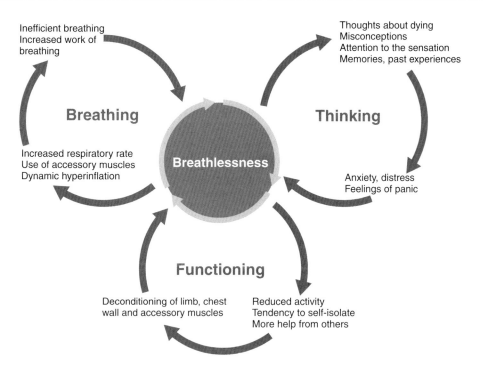

Inefficient breathing
Increased work of
breathing

Thoughts about dying
Misconceptions
Attention to the sensation
Memories, past experiences

Breathing

Thinking

Increased respiratory rate
Use of accessory muscles
Dynamic hyperinflation

Breathlessness

Anxiety, distress
Feelings of panic

Functioning

Deconditioning of limb, chest
wall and accessory muscles

Reduced activity
Tendency to self-isolate
More help from others

Figure 4.6 The Breathing, Thinking, Functioning Model

Managing Breathlessness – Break the Cycle

Fortunately, there are interventions that are effective, starting with communication.
Spathis et al. (2017) suggest some phrases to use with patients to challenge
misconceptions about breathing, thinking and functioning.

Breathing

It is natural to think that, when you are feeling breathless, you need more air
in. In fact this isn't the case – there is plenty of air in your lungs. Try instead to
lengthen your out-breath to make breathing more efficient and create space
for the next breath.

Thinking

Some people say they are terrified they are going to die gasping for breath.
This almost never happens in reality. When the time comes to die the gases
in the lung make you sleepy and calm.

Functioning

Making yourself a little more breathless doing more activity will not harm
you. In fact it strengthens the breathing muscles and will slowly improve your
general health.

In addition to challenging the misconceptions about breathlessness, there are a
number of interventions that are effective:

- **Fans** – Handheld fans are a cheap and effective intervention. Using a fan probably works by stimulating the 'diving reflex'. This reflex is present in animals that swim underwater, and originates in pre-human evolution when fish began to move onto land. The reflex stimulates facial receptors around the mouth and nose, which trigger the brain to allow breath-holding and diving underwater for prolonged periods (Schwartzstein et al., 1987). How the fan is used is critical – a brief scientific explanation of why it works and holding the fan 15–20 cm away from the face has been shown to be effective and puts a patient back in control of their breathlessness. Without an explanation the benefit is much less effective (Farquar et al., 2014).

- **Cognitive and behavioural changes** – Anxiety and breathlessness are closely linked. Functional MRI studies in breathlessness show high levels of activity in the amygdala where emotional processing occurs. This approach identifies triggers for a patient's anxiety and uses techniques to avoid them. These behavioural techniques, such as mindfulness, reduce the impact of negative thoughts (Howard and Dupont, 2014).

- **Breathing techniques** – Good breathing technique can encourage breathing control to deter hyperventilation. Pursing the lips increases airway pressure to benefit alveolar function. Blowing out during exertion and slowing the breathing with deeper breaths improves breathing control, efficiency and reduces the incidence of panic episodes.

- **Positioning and energy conservation** – Leaning forward on a table braces the upper limbs and enhances chest wall and diaphragm efficiency. Sitting forward in a chair domes the diaphragm improving ventilation efficiency (Bott et al., 2009).

Pharmacological Interventions

Opioids

This class of drugs have substantial evidence to support their use in breathlessness irrespective of the cause. Sustained-release morphine in a dose range of 10–30 mg in 24 hours produces significant effect on both the sensation of breathlessness and overall improvement in quality of life (Twycross and Wilcock, 2019). An often-cited argument against using opioids is the potential risk of respiratory depression: this is unfounded. Systematic reviews of opioid use in breathlessness have found no severe adverse effects other than constipation, which can be anticipated and managed appropriately.

The optimal dose of morphine or equivalent is still debated. Current research suggests that the higher the dose, the better the effect: 10 mg a day is effective in 30% of patients; 20 mg a day is effective in 90% of patients. The effect is patient-dependent and the current advice is to titrate the dose up using increasing doses of immediate-release morphine sulphate twice a day until an effective dose is reached. Once the effective dose is determined, the morphine can be switched to a twice-daily slow-release formulation within a range of 5–15 mg (Currow et al., 2017).

Other sustained-release opioids, such as fentanyl patches, also appear to be effective in practice, but the research evidence is currently lacking.

Benzodiazepines

This group of drugs is a widely used sedative. There has been a move towards prescribing them in chronic breathlessness, and large numbers of patients with COPD and lung cancer have them prescribed alongside opioids. However, the research evidence is clear that they have little effect on breathlessness. They do, however, have a role in panic attacks in advanced disease and can be used sublingually (Chin and Booth, 2016).

Oxygen

Huge numbers of patients with advanced COPD and lung cancer are using prescribed oxygen. There is good evidence to suggest that oxygen improves the lives of patients with hypoxia, but no evidence that it helps patients with lung cancer or COPD who are not hypoxic.

Oxygen may have a role in a small group of patients, particularly in a dying patient who has had long term oxygen and would be distressed if oxygen were to be denied. The British Thoracic Society (2006) has produced guidelines for the use of palliative oxygen therapy (POT):

- Oxygen saturation measurements **do not** correlate to the subjective sensation of breathlessness.

- Patients with hypoxia **do not** experience a significant difference in symptoms between air and POT despite the fact that saturations are improved on POT.

- Patients with mild hypoxia **do not** experience benefit with POT versus air.

- Opioids are **significantly better** than POT in reducing the intensity of breathlessness.

The lack of benefit of POT is important; oxygen is an expensive drug and a fire risk in the home. There is little evidence to support its use, and other approaches, both pharmacological and non-pharmacological, are far more effective (Hardinge, 2015). On a practical note though, removing oxygen from a patient who has become emotionally dependent on it may lead to increased calls to services and emergency department attendances.

Breathlessness in the Last Days of Life

While it is legitimate to give reassurances that patients in the dying phase are unlikely to sense breathlessness, there remains a number of patients who will become increasingly distressed by breathlessness and will need active management. If the patient is unable to swallow, a continuous subcutaneous infusion to manage restlessness, pain and nausea is indicated. A typical regimen would be:

- morphine sulphate 5–15 mg/24 hours

- midazolam 5–30 mg/24 hours

- levomepromazine 6.25–12.5 mg.

(NHS Scotland, 2019)

Key Points

- A paramedic has an important role in breathlessness management. When seeing a patient, check that all possible approaches are in place, such as fans, low-dose opioids and a benzodiazepine for panic.

- Breathlessness is a syndrome in its own right once reversible disease has been treated.

- Use the 'breathing, thinking, functioning' model as the basis for assessment and treatment.

- There is strong evidence to support a range of drug and non-drug approaches. Oxygen is not one of them.

- Cognitive approaches (such as mindfulness) effectively modify emotional responses.

- Exercise maintains function, improves quality of life and reduces social isolation. Exercise-induced breathlessness does not worsen the condition.

- At the very end of life, opioids and benzodiazepines via a syringe driver are very effective in reducing the sensation of breathlessness.

Delirium

Delirium is a common condition in the last weeks or days of life. Up to 70% of patients admitted to a specialist palliative care unit will experience delirium (Hosie et al., 2013).

Delirium is often described as an acute confusional state or agitation. Other phrases commonly employed are 'pleasantly confused', 'restless' or 'withdrawn'. All of these euphemisms are describing delirium. It is important to use the appropriate language and not dismiss this serious condition.

Regardless of the setting, anyone with delirium will have:

- a raised risk of developing dementia

- more complications in hospital, such as falls and infection

- an increased risk of ending up in long-term care

- longer hospital stays

- a significant risk of dying prematurely.

(Todd and Teale, 2017)

In a patient with advanced disease, delirium may herald the onset of dying and is often called 'terminal agitation'. A more appropriate phrase would be 'terminal or end of life delirium'.

Definition

The word delirium derives from the Latin word 'delirare' which means to 'plough across the furrow', that is, a sudden change from the normal pattern of ploughing in straight lines. This image emphasises the sudden change from normal that patients with delirium experience. Delirium is an acute brain failure and should be treated with the same urgency as any other organ failure.

Causes

Delirium is a complex condition. It occurs when acute disease impinges on a physiologically impaired brain. At the end of life, delirium is probably driven by multiple organ failure, particularly renal and hepatic failure. Disseminated intravascular coagulation, infection, drugs and hypoxia are common at the end of life and heighten the risk of delirium.

A summary of the recognised causes of delirium at end of life would include:

- **Metabolic disturbances:**
    - raised calcium, altered sodium and potassium, dehydration and altered blood sugars
- **Drugs:**
    - in particular benzodiazepines, steroids and opioids
- **Brain disorders:**
    - tumour, metastases and ischaemia
- **Sepsis and hypoxia**
- **Generalised organ failure:**
    - particularly renal and hepatic failure.
- **Constipation and urinary retention.**

High-risk factors for delirium include brain metastases, male sex, increasing age and existing cognitive impairment (Todd and Teale, 2017).

Recognising Delirium

Delirium is characterised by **incoherence, memory dysfunction** and **disorientation** which has an **acute and fluctuating** course. It develops rapidly over one to two days and is a serious condition with poor outcomes. Hallucinations may be present, such as faces on the wall or steam coming out of the floor. Many patients will have a disturbed sleep/wake cycle and have purposeless movements, such as plucking at clothes or grimacing.

Hyperactive, Hypoactive and Mixed Delirium at End of Life

Hyperactive delirium is dominated by restlessness and agitated behaviour, **hypoactive** by drowsiness and inactivity, and **mixed** delirium contains elements of both and can swing between active and hypoactive. The subtler changes of the hypoactive form are often missed. If a patient has been sitting quietly in the emergency department for five hours, and has not asked for fluids or why they are waiting, then they probably have hypoactive delirium

Screening for Delirium

There are a number of validated screening tools for delirium, which can be used alongside clinical examination and history taking. There are two tools in particular to consider adopting:

- The **4AT** (MacLullich, 2019) is a rapid and easy-to-use tool. It takes two minutes, needs no specific training and is validated in a palliative setting. The tool assesses alertness, orientation, attention and whether delirium is acute or fluctuating.

- **The Single Question in Delirium (SQUiD)** tool (McClearly and Cumming, 2015) asks one question of family or friends: 'Do you think the patient has been more confused recently?' This question separates dementia, which has a slow onset, from delirium, which is rapid. Patients with dementia who might be developing delirium can also be identified by the sudden deterioration of their cognition.

DELIRIUM – Top Tips

- **Look carefully for delirium (PINCH ME)**

  Pain

  Infection

  Constipation

  Hydration   **Then use the 4AT to help diagnose delirium**

  Medication

  Environment

- **Harness the power of the family**

  Listen to the story: when did confusion start? Use **SQUiD**: slow or rapid onset of symptoms? Encourage family to engage with management.

- **Review and stop culprit medicines**

  Amitriptyline, use of more than one analgesic, benzodiazepines and anticholinergic drugs can worsen delirium.

- **Orientate your patient**

  Clocks and calendars. Check need for hearing aids and glasses. Encourage sleep at night and not during day.

- **Avoid doing harm**

  Don't stick tubes into patients that they don't need, such as catheters and IVs.

  Don't order tests you don't routinely need such as CT head, ECGs, blood gases.

- **Delirium is not a benign condition** – it is bad news, and carries a higher risk of death, institutionalisation, prolonged hospital stays and is associated with increased risk of dementia.

- **Don't base diagnosis on a urine dip** – if a urinary tract infection is suspected send a mid-stream urine sample to the laboratory for analysis. Urine in people over 65 should not be dipped: many have asymptomatic bacteraemia and do not need treatment.
- **Don't wake patients up at night** – avoid loud noises, stop observations unless essential, don't move patients from ward to ward at night.

Adapted from information compiled by Linda Dykes (2019)

Management

The management of delirium involves a range of positive measures; there are a number of interventions that should be avoided as they can make the situation worse.

In a palliative care inpatient setting, any treatment will be focused on conditions that might be reversible, e.g. infection or hypercalcaemia. Up to 50% of delirium is reversible in a hospital setting but results are significantly lower in hospices (Caraceni and Grassi, 2003). At all times this is done in context – where is the patient in the progression of their disease? What would be their views on treating reversible conditions? Many patients will have expressed clear ceilings of care in anticipation of acute episodes, and it is the duty of all professionals to abide by these. To recover a patient from an acute episode of delirium for them to die a few days later may not be in a patient's or family's wishes or best interests.

Drug Therapy

Drug therapy in delirium is aimed at reducing agitation and perceptual abnormalities such as hallucinations. This is a difficult area; the most recent Cochrane review made no drug recommendations for managing delirium at end of life (Burry et al., 2018). Palliative care was specifically excluded from the NICE guidelines on delirium, so drug approaches are pragmatic, experience based and not evidenced. NICE recommends haloperidol as the drug of choice outside a palliative setting (NICE, 2019). This drug is widely adopted by palliative teams, however, particularly if hallucinations are a prominent feature. Haloperidol has significant issues, particularly extrapyramidal side effects in older patients, and benzodiazepines, such as midazolam, are used in preference (Hosker and Bennett, 2016).

A recent randomised double blind trial of antipsychotics and placebo in delirium showed that antipsychotics such as haloperidol cause significant side effects and that patients treated with placebo had a better survival rate (Agar et al., 2017). The patients in this paper had mild to moderate symptoms and the drug doses used were relatively low. How far this conclusion can be applied to a typical inpatient unit is difficult to judge. What is clear though is that antipsychotic drugs have significant side effects and should be used with caution.

In an inpatient palliative unit, patients near to death with refractory delirium may need very large doses of sedation. The drugs used are often a mixture of high doses of midazolam and levomepromazine; if that fails then third-line drugs, such as phenobarbitone, are added (Hosker and Bennet, 2016).

The Effects of Delirium on Families

The ethical issues around the use of sedation in palliative care are outside of this chapter's scope; however, it is important to stress that sedation must be used appropriately and in discussion with the wider palliative team. It should always be discussed with family or friends.

Delirium can be very stressful for families. Finucane et al. (2017) outlines the impact and helplessness families experience when witnessing delirium. Without explanation, families can jump to the conclusion that the treatments, such as analgesics, are causing the problem. While that will have an element of truth, the key issue is that the underlying disease is the primary cause. Discuss the causes and the implications, especially if the relative is entering the last few days of life. A clear explanation will be of great benefit for a family, reduce complaints and misunderstandings, and help the bereavement process when the patient dies.

Key Points

- Look for delirium and call it delirium – avoid euphemisms such as 'confusion'.
- Is there an advance care plan that might guide how the patient should be managed if capacity is lost?
- Explain to families what they are seeing and reassure that this can be managed.
- Simple things matter – look for glasses or hearing aids and ensure a quiet calming atmosphere.

Respiratory Secretions at End of Life

Noisy respiratory secretions (NRS) occur in 30–50% of patients at the end of their lives. It is often referred to as the 'death rattle' and this description is apt as the onset of the noises in an unconscious patient usually indicates that death will occur within hours to short days (Lokker et al., 2014).

Causes

Saliva in the upper airway combined with a reduced swallowing reflex is the most common reason for NRS. Lung inflammation from infection, gastric reflux and pulmonary oedema are also frequent causes.

Explaining to Patient's Family

NRS are disturbing for both families and healthcare workers. There can be pressure from families to 'do something', though some evidence suggests that healthcare workers sometimes treat secretions in the assumption that families are distressed, when in reality they are not. As far as can be determined, an unconscious patient will be unaware of NRS and explaining that to families can be the most effective treatment.

Management

Non-pharmacological approaches are usually effective. Sitting the patient upright (particularly if pulmonary oedema is suspected) or in a semi-prone position may reduce the noise. Suction is very rarely used and only in an unconscious patient.

Pharmacological approaches involve using either glycopyrronium or hyoscine butylbromide (Buscopan). However, once secretions are established, there is no evidence to show that NRS are reduced with anti-secretory medications. In practice though, these drugs are widely used and, if employed before secretions are established, they may have a role.

If the decision is made to start treatment, give an SC dose of glycopyrronium 200–400 micrograms and set up a continuous subcutaneous infusion of 600–1200 micrograms over 24 hours (Twycross and Wilcock, 2018).

If NRS is caused by respiratory tract infection, there is no role for antibiotics in reducing purulent secretions. In pulmonary oedema, diuretics such as furosemide 20–40 mg given subcutaneously or intravenously may help (Twycross and Wilcock, 2018).

Urinary Retention

Beware of urinary retention in a dying patient. Anti-secretory medication can cause retention, and inserting a catheter in a dying patient is often necessary, and essential if diuretics are used in pulmonary oedema.

Key Points

- Relatives are often distressed by NRS.
- Explain why they occur.
- Explain this is a normal part of dying.
- Reassure that, as far as we can tell, the patient will be unaware of NRS.
- Try repositioning first, then offer a pharmacological approach if appropriate.

Constipation

Constipation is the infrequent passing of stools or passing hard, painful stools. It is common in the general population and very common in patients admitted to hospices. In the last few days to weeks of life up to a half of patients admit to constipation. Constipation is a significant problem and can lead to pain, bowel obstruction, overflow diarrhoea, urinary retention and delirium (Larkin et al., 2008).

Causes

- **Disease** – Advancing disease and frailty can reduce mobility and food intake. Poor mobility restricts access to toilets, loss of appetite reduces the bulk and fibre content of food. Nausea and vomiting lower fluid and food intake, and cancer-induced weakness can affect abdominal muscles, lowering the ability to raise intra-abdominal pressure and defecate.

- **Medication** – Opioids are a major contributor to constipation. By attaching to receptors in the bowel wall they reduce peristalsis and stool transit. Opioid patches are less constipating and are an alternative route of analgesia (Camilleri and Bharucha, 2010). Other drugs, such as diuretics, lower fluid in the bowel and stools become harder. Antiemetics, particularly ondansetron and granisetron, are both 5-HT$_3$ antagonists; their effect in the bowel is to reduce transit time and harden stools.

History and Examination

Ask about recent bowel movements:

- What has changed in terms of frequency and type of stool?
- When was the last bowel movement?
- Are there any abdominal symptoms, such as colic, nausea or vomiting?
- What laxatives are being used?
- What medication is the patient taking?

Examine the abdomen:

- Are bowel sounds normal?
- Is the bowel obstructed?
- Are there any masses to palpate?

Examine the rectum (if within the clinical competencies of the paramedic attending):

- Is it full of stools or empty?

Consider screening blood for hypercalcaemia and thyroid disease.

Management

Constipation is best managed as a team with the aim of improving mobility (physiotherapy), access to toilets (occupational therapy micro-environment) and dietician.

Rectal Treatments

Rectal measures are not first-line management for constipation; oral treatments at high doses should be tried first.

Treatment depends on rectal findings:

- If the stools are hard, soften with glycerine suppositories.
- If the stools are soft, stimulate rectal expulsion with bisacodyl suppositories.

Enemas can be helpful, particularly arachis oil if inserted and left overnight (**NB**: not to be used if the patient has a nut allergy).

Key Points

- Constipation is a common cause of symptoms.
- Most patients on opioids need a regular laxative (Table 4.4) – has this been prescribed?
- Can the patient swallow? If not, switch to a rectal treatment such as suppositories.
- If taking a macrogol, can the patient manage the large volumes of fluid needed?
- Patches are less constipating than oral opioids – consider switching if constipation is resistant to treatment.

Table 4.4 Drug therapies: laxatives

Class	Example	Action	Comments
Osmotic	Lactulose	Draws water into gut by osmosis – increased volume and peristalsis	Can cause cramps and distension
Macrogols	Laxido, movicol	Drunk with large volume of water, macrogols are not absorbed – increased volume and peristalsis	Useful for faecal impaction if patient can manage large volumes of fluid
Surfactants	Docusate	Increases the amount of water absorbed by the stool	Mainly used as a stool softener
Stimulants	Senna, bisacodyl	Activated by bacteria in the large bowel to stimulate peristalsis	Can cause colic; avoid if obstruction suspected
Peripheral opioid antagonists	Methylnaltrexone, naloxegol	Displaces opioid in the gut, restores peristalsis. The drug of last resort when all other methods have failed	Can work rapidly; does not affect opioid receptors elsewhere, pain relief from opioid continues

(Adapted from NHS Scotland, 2019)

Hiccups

Hiccups can be a very troublesome symptom and one that is difficult to palliate. Hiccups is common in the general population, is usually short lived and often an item of fun. At the end of life small things become important, particularly communication and eating. Intractable hiccups can remove both these pleasures.

As with all symptoms, good history taking and examination may point to a cause. However, despite a large number of research studies there is little evidence to support the many treatments used.

Assessment

When assessing hiccups consider the following:

- Consider the **duration** and **impact** of hiccups on the patient's quality of life.

- **Gastric stasis** and distension of the abdomen is the most common cause.

- **Reflux disease** from hiatus hernia or outflow obstruction.

- **Renal failure and other metabolic diseases**, such as hypercalcaemia, can produce intractable hiccups.

- **Hepatic distension** and damage to the phrenic nerve, as well as diaphragm irritation from ascites or tumour, are also common causes.

- **Raised intracranial pressure** from brain metastases can trigger hiccups via the phrenic nerve.

Management

Simple measures can help. Drinking ice cold water, drinking small volumes of vinegar (or squirting up the nose!) and breath holding during a hiccup are commonly used. Drinking from the opposite/wrong side of the cup and rubbing the soft palate with a swab is also advocated.

In specific causes the following approaches can be tried:

- **Reflux disease** – high dose proton pump inhibitors (e.g. lansoprazole) with an antacid

- **Gastric stasis** – prokinetic drugs (e.g. metoclopramide, domperidone or erythromycin)

- **Renal/hepatic failure** – antipsychotics (e.g. haloperidol)

- **Diaphragmatic irritation** – refer for drainage of ascites if present; try a steroid (e.g. dexamethasone)

- **Intracranial pressure** – high doses of dexamethasone (Twycross and Wilcock, 2018).

Intractable Hiccups

The cause of hiccups is often multifactorial and resistant to 'cause-specific' treatment. In specialist units a wide range of drugs are used 'off licence' to manage hiccups. These drugs include calcium antagonists (e.g. nifedipine), pregabalin and baclofen (Twycross and Wilcock, 2018).

Key Points

- Hiccups are relatively common at end of life.
- The evidence for treatments is sparse.
- Try simple measures; they often help.
- A lot of patients buy peppermint water. This should not be taken with a prokinetic such as metoclopramide, as it opposes the effect on the gastro-oesophageal sphincter.
- Involve a local palliative team if treatments fail, especially if hiccups are affecting sleep.

Case Studies

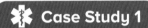 **Case Study 1**

Jane is a 56-year-old woman who attended the emergency department at a weekend with acute lower thoracic back pain. In the previous few weeks she had noted that her weight was going down and she felt generally unwell. Her only other symptom was mild epigastric discomfort. The pain had started the day before and rapidly worsened. She describes the severity as 9/10 (the only pain she had encountered that was worse was childbirth). The pain was burning, stinging and felt like an electric current in her back.

An x-ray showed no abnormality.

She was started on a 12 microgram/hour fentanyl patch and told this was the lowest dose patch and therefore a small dose. Jane has not had opiates before.

She was discharged home and told to see her GP on Monday morning.

- What type of pain is Jane describing?
- Comment on the dose of the patch: is this a low dose? (Use an opioid conversion app or chart)

Jane was seen on Monday by a paramedic attached to a GP surgery. The paramedic noted that Jane was drowsy and incoherent.

- What signs and symptoms would suggest that Jane is opioid toxic?

The paramedic is concerned by the history of weight loss and epigastric pain. An urgent CT scan is arranged, which confirms a pancreatic cancer.

- Why did the pain initially occur in Jane's back?
- What class of drugs would you use to control the pain other than opioids?
- Jane's patch is stopped and she commences morphine sulphate MR (modified-release) 15 mg twice a day. What would the pro re nata (PRN) breakthrough dose of morphine sulphate IR (instant-release) be?

🔯 Case Study 2

John is a 75-year-old man with chronic obstructive pulmonary disease. He frequently calls his GP and the 999 service complaining of acute shortness of breath. He has had frequent courses of antibiotics and steroids, often prescribed over the phone as he is so well known to the local practice. He says they make no difference.

A paramedic team is dispatched late one night. On arrival they find John panting for breath. His oxygen saturations are near normal. The only drugs in the house are a 'rescue course' of steroids and antibiotics.

- Why might John be short of breath?
- John says he always gets oxygen when this happens. Would oxygen be an appropriate treatment?
- The paramedics conclude John is getting episodes of panic and he is referred back to his GP for management. What might the GP do to manage John's symptoms?

A week later a further call is received late at night. John is complaining of acute shortness of breath. In the house the paramedics find a handheld fan, a box of oxazepam and a bottle of morphine sulphate IR. John said the fan didn't work and he feared he would stop breathing if he took opiates.

- Is there evidence that fans work for breathlessness? What instructions could you give to John that have been shown to make fans more effective?
- Is John correct in thinking that opiates suppress the respiratory centre?
- A distinct syndrome of chronic breathlessness has been described in the literature. What are the three areas that need to be addressed to manage John's symptoms?

✚ Case Study 3

Anne is a 40-year-old woman with advanced ovarian cancer. A recent scan shows widespread tumour across the peritoneum. Anne asks for a home visit as she started to vomit and feels unwell.

- What is the difference between nausea and vomiting?
- What are the possible causes of Anne's symptoms?
- What investigations might be undertaken?

Anne is examined and she has a tender abdomen, has not opened her bowels for 48 hours but is passing flatus. Anne says she eats a small amount and feels full immediately.

- Which antiemetic might help Anne's symptoms and why?

Anne's blood test comes back and she has a high calcium and a low sodium.

- Which antiemetic might be used for vomiting due to chemical causes?

Anne develops new symptoms and has a CT scan of her head, which shows cerebral metastases.

- Which antiemetic is commonly used for vomiting caused by raised intracranial pressure?
- What are the physiological events that happen almost simultaneously to produce vomiting?

✚ Case Study 4

Albert is an 88-year-old man who has been admitted to a palliative care unit. He has widespread bone metastases from prostate cancer. He has a bag full of drugs including two antihypertensives, oral morphine, a diuretic and codeine. Unfortunately, his daughter was unable to accompany him to the unit. The nurses observe that he is deaf, appears very withdrawn, plucking at the bed sheets, and told one of the nurses that there are faces in the curtains.

- How would you try and determine whether Albert has dementia or delirium?
- What one question might you ask his daughter on the phone?

Julie, Albert's daughter, visits and more history is taken. Julie says that Albert has had a slow but steady decline in his memory, but suddenly changed and became withdrawn and hallucinating. His pain had worsened and he was 'swigging morphine' most of the day. The ward team consider Albert has delirium.

- What type of delirium is Albert experiencing?
- List the possible triggers for Albert's delirium?
- What would be your management plan?

All the drugs are stopped and Albert emerges from the delirium. He spends two weeks on the unit and is clearly dying. One night he starts shouting out and throwing items from his bedside table. He is very distressed and rolling around in the bed.

- What type of delirium is he exhibiting?
- What might be a cause for this sudden deterioration? What physical examination might help find the cause?

Further Reading

National Institute for Health and Care Excellence (2017). *End of Life Care for Adults* (QS13). London: NICE. Available at: https://www.nice.org.uk/guidance/qs13.

Watson S et al. (2019). *Oxford Handbook of Palliative Care* (3rd ed.). Oxford: Oxford Medical Handbooks.

The Palliative Adult Network Guidelines Plus is a comprehensive resource and is available on open access at: https://book.pallcare.info/.

The Royal College of GPs *Palliative and End of Life Care Toolkit*: https://www.rcgp.org.uk/clinical-and-research/resources/toolkits/palliative-and-end-of-life-care-toolkit.aspx.

Marie Curie have extensive resources for both patients and professionals: https://www.mariecurie.org.uk/help.

The BNF has helpful sections on controlled drugs and prescribing in palliative care: https://www.bnf.org/.

Local hospices will have guidelines on their website together with contact numbers.

Paramedics in general practice or hospital settings are encouraged to join a college such as the Royal College of General Practitioners or Royal College of Physicians in addition to the College of Paramedics. Colleges will have access to extensive resources on palliative care. The College of Paramedics run palliative care courses on communication skills and symptom management. For up-to-date information visit their website: https://www.collegeofparamedics.co.uk/.

References

Agar MR et al. (2017). Efficacy of oral risperidone, haloperidol, or placebo for symptoms of delirium among patients in palliative care: a randomized clinical trial. *JAMA Internal Medicine*, 177(1): 34–42.

Ashley C and Currie A (2019). *The Renal Drug Handbook*. Available at: https://www.pharmalink.nl/docs/renalbook.pdf.

BNF (2019). *British National Formulary*, (77th ed.). Nottingham: Pharmaceutical Press.

Booth S, Chin C and Spathis A (2015). The brain and breathlessness: understanding and disseminating a palliative care approach. *Palliative Medicine*, 29(5): 396–398.

Bott J et al. (2009). Guidelines for the physiotherapy management of the adult, medical, spontaneously breathing patient. *Thorax*, 64(1): i1–i52.

British Thoracic Society (2006). *Working Group on Home Oxygen Services. Clinical Component for the Home Oxygen Service in England and Wales*. London: BTS.

Buckley N, Dawson A and Isbister G (2014). Serotonin syndrome. *BMJ*, 348: g1626.

Burry L et al. (2018). Antipsychotics for treatment of delirium in hospitalised non-ICU patients. *Cochrane Database of Systematic Reviews*, 6: CD005594.

Camilleri M and Bharucha A (2010). Behavioural and new pharmacological treatments for constipation: getting the balance right. *Gut*, 59(9): 1288–1296.

Caraceni L and Grassi A (2003). Delirium and acute confusional states in palliative medicine. *Supportive Care in Cancer*, 11(11): 745.

Carlson CL (2016). Effectiveness of the World Health Organization cancer pain relief guidelines: an integrative review. *Journal of Pain Research*, 9: 515–534.

Chin C and Booth S (2016) Managing breathlessness: a palliative care approach. *Postgraduate Medical Journal*, 92(1089): 393.

Currow D et al. (2010). Do the trajectories of dyspnoea differ in prevalence and intensity by diagnosis at the end of life? A consecutive cohort study. *Journal of Pain and Symptom Management*, 39(4): 680–690.

Currow D et al. (2017). A pragmatic, phase III, multisite, double-blind, placebo-controlled, parallel-arm, dose increment randomised trial of regular, low-dose extended-release morphine for chronic breathlessness: breathlessness, exertion and morphine sulfate (BEAMS) study protocol. *BMJ Open*, 7(7): e018100.

DisDAT Tool: Northumberland Tyne & Wear NHS Trust and St. Oswald's Hospice (2006). *Disability Distress Assessment Tool*. Northumberland: St Oswald's Hospice. Available at: https://www.stoswaldsuk.org/how-we-help/we-educate/education/resources/disability-distress-assessment-tool-disdat/disdat-tools/.

Dykes L (2019). *Dr Linda Dykes: Medical Education Resources*. Available at: https://www.lindadykes.org/.

Farquhar MC et al. (2014). Is a specialist breathlessness service more effective and cost-effective for patients with advanced cancer and their carers than standard care? Findings of a mixed-method randomised controlled trial. *BMC Medicine*, 12: 194.

Finnerup NB et al. (2015). Pharmacotherapy for neuropathic pain in adults: a systematic review and meta-analysis. *The Lancet. Neurology*, 14(2): 162–173.

Finucane A, Lugton J and Kennedy CJ (2017). The experiences of caregivers of patients with delirium, and their role in its management in palliative care settings: an integrative literature review. *Psycho-Oncology*, 26(3): 291–300.

Hardinge M et al. (2015). British Thoracic Society guidelines for home oxygen use in adults: accredited by NICE. *Thorax*, 70(1): i1-i43.

Harris D (2010). Nausea and vomiting in advanced cancer. *British Medical Bulletin*, 96(1): 175–185.

Hosie A et al. (2013). Delirium prevalence, incidence, and implications for screening in specialist palliative care inpatient settings: a systematic review. *Palliative Medicine*, 27(6): 486–498.

Hosker C and Bennett M (2016). Delirium and agitation at the end of life. *BMJ*, 353(3): i3085.

Howard C and Dupont S (2014). 'The COPD breathlessness manual': a randomised controlled trial to test a cognitive-behavioural manual versus information booklets on health service use, mood and health status, in patients with chronic obstructive pulmonary disease. *NPJ Primary Care Respiratory Medicine*, 24: 14076.

Johnson M and Yorke J (2017). Towards an expert consensus to delineate a clinical syndrome of chronic breathlessness. *European Respiratory Journal*, 49: 1602277.

Jordan A (2011). The utility of PAINAD in assessing pain in a UK population with severe dementia. *European Journal of Geriatric Psychiatry*, 26(2): 118–126.

Larkin P et al. (2008). The management of constipation in palliative care: clinical practice recommendations. *Palliative Medicine*, 22(7): 796–807.

Leeds Community Healthcare and St Gemma's Hospice (2016). *The Leeds Opioid Conversion Guide for Adult Palliative Care Patients*. Available at: http://www.cpwy.org/doc/1273.pdf.

Leppert W and Luczak J (2005). The role of tramadol in cancer pain treatment – a review. *Support Care Cancer*, 13(1): 5–7.

Lokker I et al. (2014). Prevalence, impact, and treatment of death rattle: a systematic review. *Journal of Pain and Symptom Management*, 47(1): 105–122.

MacLullich A (2019). *4AT Rapid Clinical Test for Delirium*. Available at: www.the4AT.com.

McCaffery M (1994). *Pain: Clinical Manual for Nursing Practice*. London: Mosby.

McClearly E and Cumming P (2015). Improving early recognition delirium using SQiD (Single question to identify delirium). *BMJ Open Quality*, 4(1).

Mehta A and Chan LS (2008) Understanding the concept of 'Total Pain': a prerequisite for pain control. *Journal of Hospice and Palliative Nursing*, 10(1): 26–32.

MRC (2008). *Breathlessness Scale*. Available at: https://mrc.ukri.org/research/facilities-and-resources-for-researchers/mrc-scales/mrc-dyspnoea-scale-mrc-breathlessness-scale/.

NHS Scotland (2019). *Scottish Palliative Care Guidelines*. Available at: https://www.palliativecareguidelines.scot.nhs.uk/.

National Institute for Health and Care Excellence (2012). *Palliative care for adults: strong opioids for pain relief [CG140]*. Available at: https://www.nice.org.uk/guidance/cg140/chapter/1-Recommendations#first-line-treatment-if-oral-opioids-are-not-suitable-transdermal-patches.

National Institute for Health and Care Excellence (2019). *Delirium: Prevention, Diagnosis and Management* (CG103). Available at: https://www.nice.org.uk/guidance/CG103.

Saunders C (1964). The symptomatic treatment of incurable malignant disease. *Prescribers Journal*, 4(4): 68–73.

Saunders C (1970). Nature and management of terminal pain. In Shotter, E. (ed.), *Matters of Life and Death*. London: Dartman, Longman & Todd: 15–26.

Schwartzstein RM et al. (1987). Cold facial stimulation reduces breathlessness induced in normal subjects. *American Review of Respiratory Disease*, 136: 58–61.

SCIE – Social Care Institute for Excellence (2019). *Decision Making Capacity in Dementia*. Available at: https://www.scie.org.uk/dementia/supporting-people-with-dementia/decisions/capacity.asp.

Smith T and Saiki C (2015). Cancer pain management. *Mayo Clinic Proceedings*, 90(10): 1428–1439.

Spathis A et al. (2017). The Breathing, Thinking, Functioning clinical model: a proposal to facilitate evidence-based breathlessness management in chronic respiratory disease. *Nature Partner Journals Primary Care Respiratory Medicine*, 27(1): 27.

Stephenson J and Davies A (2006). An assessment of aetiology-based guidelines for the management of nausea and vomiting in patients with advanced cancer. *Supportive Care in Cancer*, 14(4): 348–353.

Thomas J and Monaghan T (2014). *Oxford Handbook of Clinical Examination and Practical Skills* (2nd ed.). Oxford: Oxford Medical Handbooks.

Todd O and Teale E (2017). Delirium: a guide for the general physician. *Clinical Medicine (London, England)*, 17(1): 48–53.

Treede R, Rief W and Barke A (2015). A classification of chronic pain for ICD-11. *Pain*, 156(6): 1003–1007.

Twycross R and Wilcock A (2018) *Introducing Palliative Care* (5th ed.) Nottingham: Pharmaceutical Press.

Twycross R and Wilcock A (2019). *PCF6 Palliative Care Formulary* (6th ed.) Nottingham: Pharmaceutical Press.

Watson M et al. (2020). *Palliative Care Adult Network Guidelines*. Available at: https://book.pallcare. info/.

World Health Organization (1986). *Cancer Pain Relief: With a Guide to Opioid Availability* (2nd ed.). Geneva: WHO.

Wood H et al. (2018) Updates in palliative care – overview and recent advancements in the pharmacological management of cancer pain. *Clinical Medicine*, 18(1): 17–22.

Chapter 5

Enhanced Communication Skills in Palliative and End of Life Care

Alison Rae

Introduction

The National Institute for Health and Care Excellence (NICE) guidance for supportive and palliative care in cancer services (NICE, 2004) emphasises the value of effective communication. Furthermore, Health Education England (2017) have developed an end of life care core skills education and training framework, which supports the notion that communication is at the heart of every aspect of end of life care. However, there seem to be a number of barriers that can affect the delivery of clear communication, especially at the time of patient death (Rodenbach et al., 2016). Common communication difficulties include illnesses that can cause dysarthria (difficulty speaking), learning disability, sensory impairment, and if the patient does not speak the same language as the healthcare provider (Marie Curie, 2019). Other barriers include time constraints, competing demands, interruptions and environmental factors. Health professionals may also feel awkward about talking to complete strangers about very difficult issues (Ali, 2017).

Paramedics are required to communicate with patients facing death and this part of their role can be extremely daunting for some practitioners, so effective training in enhanced communication skills is vital. They may feel anxious, tense, emotionally challenged and unable to provide effective care. Part of the reason why clinicians in general find communication with terminally ill patients difficult is due to their own unexamined attitudes towards death (Rodenbach et al., 2016). If a person has not accepted their own mortality, they are more likely to focus on biomedical issues rather than a dying patient's emotional needs (Rodenbach et al., 2016). To address this in practice, paramedics need to first explore their own opinions about death. Once they understand and make sense of their individual feelings or beliefs, and are no longer restricted by fear or apprehension, they will be better placed to learn new and effective ways of communicating with palliative and end of life patients, their relatives and friends.

Allowing patients to have a good death requires skilled communication as well as advanced medical treatment (Higgins, 2010). As healthcare professionals it is necessary for paramedics to consider how people cope with the dying process, and in what manner their psychological, spiritual and physical needs can be best addressed. The NICE guidance on *Improving Supportive and Palliative Care for Adults with Cancer* (2004) highlights the value of effective communication as a way of providing emotional support and championing informed decision making at the end of life. The guidance also recommends that all healthcare professionals should be taught advanced communication skills.

Learning and trying out new ways of communicating can be unnerving, but it is necessary to ensure that any exchange of information is as effective as possible. Arguably, it is an emerging component of the paramedic role to accurately determine each patient's hopes and aspirations in terms of the death they would like to have. Furthermore, with an increasing number of palliative care patients remaining at home, paramedics are likely to receive an increase in the number of emergency calls from relatives who are acting as caregivers when situations deteriorate and there is an immediate need for information and advice (Wiese et al., 2009).

To assist paramedics in developing their individual communication skills, this chapter will focus primarily on the following elements:

- Communication with patients, family and friends
- Advocating for patients
- Communicating with other professional
- Breaking bad news
- Telling the truth in clinical practice
- Referrals, documentation and follow-up
- Hope and communication.

Communication with Patients, Family and Friends

Effective communication is central to fostering high-quality care at the end of life (Kinghorn et al., 2007). While advanced communication skills take practice, time, desire and motivation to be learnt (Richardson, 2018), poor communication can cause patients and their families further anxiety and fear and exacerbate the physical symptoms associated with their underlying pathology. What patients tend to need at the end of life is communication that is honest, sensitive to their needs, reassuring and informative.

Pause for thought

There is a strong and definite need for paramedics to independently consider what makes a good death. This can be achieved by writing a list of things they personally would like to achieve or affairs they wish to put in order before they die. This type of task helps individuals to focus on what would be important to them thus leading to a truer sense of empathy with patients who are actually at this junction in their lives.

The qualities of a good communicator include the ability to receive and interpret messages, to listen with the intent to understand the individual needs of each person, and to make allowances where necessary (Kozlowska and Doboszynska, 2012). A good communicator is also able to manage barriers such as cultural or language differences, as well as compromised cognitive and emotional states (Webb, 2011). A patient-centred approach is essential, using language that is clear, unambiguous and free from medical jargon (Wittenberg-Lyles et al., 2013).

Communication can be performed in two ways: verbally (with words) and non-verbally (without words) (Kozlowska and Doboszynska, 2012). In terms of non-verbal communication, it is important for healthcare professionals to always adopt a posture that invites discussion, i.e. avoiding crossed arms (Kuebler et al., 2007). Other non-verbal strategies include giving the patient undivided attention, directly facing the patient at their eye level, leaning forwards and being self-aware, and avoiding distracting mannerisms, e.g. over-exaggerated hand gestures (Moore, 2005). The tone of voice is important too, ensuring the one adopted is not patronising or demeaning. This will demonstrate empathy and sympathy, while recognising that no one individual will feel the same way. Verbal behaviours might include avoiding interruptions (by putting mobile phones on silent), establishing the patient's beliefs, values and desires, providing information, checking understanding and offering reassurance and support.

It is important to remember that how people die remains in the memory of those who live on. So the correct and sensitive management of the family during the dying process is extremely important. Decision making, especially in relation to family-witnessed resuscitation, can be a central issue to some paramedics. Where families cannot handle the emotion of witnessed resuscitation, it is described as an inappropriate course of action, as it exacerbates their distress (Waldrop et al., 2015). Careful consideration to initiating resuscitation in the first place is also necessary, as CPR can reverse the dying process. If the patient has chosen a dignified death and mortality is expected, then the patient should be issued with a correctly completed Do Not Attempt Cardiopulmonary Resuscitation (DNACPR) decision/order so that CPR is not necessary if families call emergency services at the time of death.

Attempted cardiopulmonary resuscitation or CPR is rarely successful for patients who have been deteriorating over previous weeks (Miller and Dorman, 2014). In fact, one study found that none of the 171 patients with cancer who had a cardiorespiratory arrest after a period of deterioration, survived (Ewer et al., 2001). Interestingly, patients who have dementia alongside their cancer diagnosis are also likely to have a poor outcome (Ebell et al., 1998).

When patients have a completed DNACPR order or decision but the document cannot be located, pre-hospital providers should still start resuscitation, even if the family state that the patient did not want it (Waldrop et al., 2015). For further guidance on circumstances where paramedics may stop or not resuscitate please refer to the JRCALC guidelines 2019 (JRCALC, 2019: 'Validation of DNACPR' on page 114). If the family of the patient disagree with the commencement of CPR this can cause conflict and have a detrimental effect on everyone involved. To address this issue in part, a new process called ReSPECT creates personalised recommendations for a person's clinical care in a future emergency in which they are unable to make or express their own choices. It has been developed following the results of a systematic review in 2014 of DNACPR decisions presented by a team from Warwick University at the Royal Society of Medicine. The ReSPECT form is a summary plan that records recommendations to guide clinical decision making but it is not a legally binding document.

The ethical and legal principles that underpin best practice in decisions relating to CPR by the British Medical Association, Resuscitation Council (UK) and Royal College of Nursing are valid for the ReSPECT process. Ultimately decisions relating to CPR promote more advance planning, good communication, shared decision making and excellent documentation (ReSPECT, 2017). Further guidance on CPR provision has been published by the General Medical Council (2010).

Barriers to Communication: FEARS/FIBS

There are clear barriers to effective communication, which can exist either on the part of the patient/family member or the healthcare professional (Nicol and Nyatanga, 2017). These barriers can take many guises, for example patients who have a sensory impairment, such as poor hearing or sight. However, there are simple strategies one can use, such as ensuring patients are wearing their hearing aids or glasses (Nicol and Nyatanga, 2017). Where a patient lacks decision-making capacity, there are a number of ways that decisions can be reached on the patient's behalf, such as a valid advance decision to refuse a specified treatment (ADRT) (Nicol and Nyatanga, 2017). However, there are a number of conditions that must be satisfied for an ADRT to be valid (Department for Constitutional Affairs, 2007).

Potential clinician barriers that will interfere with effective communication include a lack of awareness of the plan of care, time constraints and lack of continuity of care. It is best practice to always ask to see existing care plans. Ensure they have been recently reviewed by the relevant healthcare professionals and that everything has been carried out in accordance with the plan. Try to make eye contact with patients and don't avoid answering their difficult questions (Maguire et al., 1996). Always ask the patient how they are feeling; check to see if they are in pain and if this is the same pain or worse than before. Unrelieved pain can be an enormous barrier to effective communication causing depression and anxiety and distress (Farrer, 2007).

There are two useful frameworks that have been developed to support healthcare professionals in recognising and addressing barriers to effective communication. The first is represented by the acronym FEARS (fears, environment, attitudes, responses, skills) and the second by the acronym FIBS (fears, inadequate skills, beliefs, support) (Nicol and Nyatanga, 2017). These frameworks are shown in Tables 5.1 and 5.2.

Table 5.1 FEARS: potential patient barriers to communication

FEARS Element	Manifestation
Fears	Being judged as ungrateful; being stigmatised; crying/breaking down; burdening/causing distress to the health professional
Environment	Lack of privacy; person present or absent who needs to be/not be there with me
Attitudes	This person does not have time to listen to me, or it is not this person's job to talk about this; my concerns are not important; I should be able to cope with this; my family would not want me to talk about this
Responses (from healthcare professionals)	Distanced or disengaged; relevant questions were not asked of me; being touched when I need my own space
Skills	I cannot find the right words/have not sufficient command of language/do not understand enough to know what to ask; literacy levels; mental capacity issues

(Nicol and Nyatanga, 2017: 36)

Table 5.2 FIBS: potential barriers to communication

FIBS Element	Manifestation
Fears	Causing upset or harm; emotional responses; saying 'the wrong thing'; being asked difficult questions; taking too much time
Inadequate skills	Lack of assessment skills for psychological issues and concerns as well as physical ones; inability to integrate physical and non-physical agenda together into a full holistic review
Beliefs	Emotional problems are inevitable in serious/life-threatening illness nothing can be done about them so it is pointless to bring up issues we 'cannot solve'; it is 'someone else's role to do this'
Support	Lack of support for the patient if problems are identified; feeling professionally unsupported; team conflicts

(Nicol and Nyatanga, 2017: 36)

Consider Your Own Practice

Paramedics considering their own practice may find it helpful to discuss their fears and concerns with colleagues or other members of the multidisciplinary team. Clinical supervision is one way of achieving this. Clinical supervision is a framework used by healthcare professionals to maintain and develop standards of care, focusing on self-awareness and development (Davenport, 2013). It is important to remember that if practitioners do not manage their own barriers, they will not be able to effectively communicate with others. Self-awareness will support success in this endeavour, along with a focus on patient-centred care and shared decision making. *No Decisions About Me Without Me* captures the true spirit of this message (Coulter and Collins, 2011).

Penrod et al. (2011) found three end of life trajectories: expected death (where patients decline rapidly), unexpected death (where patients decline slowly, then suddenly experience an exacerbation of symptoms that lead to a quick death) and mixed death (comprising both of the previous elements). Where symptoms are unexpected and/or exacerbations unanticipated, family or caregivers make calls to emergency services that can sometimes result in death before arrival to hospital, pre-hospital resuscitation or terminal decline (Waldrop et al., 2015). As a result, emergency calls are often made when patients reach the end of their lives because they start to suffer with alarming symptoms, such as noisy and laboured breathing; family and care givers panic and paramedics will be the professionals they reach out to for help and reassurance.

Watching someone die, with or without active resuscitative attempts, can be extremely difficult for some people to cope with (Waldrop et al., 2015). However, for end of life choices to be upheld and supported by attending paramedics, they may need to silence their own opinions and know when to advocate for patients.

Patient Advocacy

A patient advocate can be defined as a person who helps a patient work with others who influence their health. This help typically involves resolving issues around healthcare (National Cancer Institute, 2017). Trevithick (2012) suggests that advocacy aims to ensure that the patient's voice is heard, giving them greater say in how they live their lives and the services they need to help them do so. Although this may sound like a simple concept, it can be complex, especially for paramedics who may be attending a patient out of area, so are not familiar with the local services available.

All healthcare professionals have a legal responsibility to ensure that any acts or omissions do not cause harm to anyone (Nicol and Nyatanga, 2017). Bateman (1995) also suggests that there are six main principles when implementing patient advocacy. These include: acting in the client's best interests and in accordance with their wishes; keeping the client properly informed at all times; carrying out instructions with diligence and competence; acting impartially; offering independent and frank advice; and finally, maintaining confidentiality.

There are other factors to consider when acting as an advocate, including the mental capacity of the patient. In palliative care a person who has been previously competent may be less so due to the disease process, medications and decreasing consciousness (Kinghorn et al., 2007). Where the patient lacks decision-making capacity there are alternative ways in which decisions can be made on their behalf (Nicol and Nyatanga, 2017). Under the *Mental Capacity Act 2005* the patient may have made a valid advance decision to refuse a specified treatment (ADRT). If paramedics identify an applicable and valid ADRT then they will be protected from legal liability for withdrawing or withholding treatment. However, a number of conditions must be fulfilled for an ADRT to be valid (for more information, please refer to the Department of Constitutional Affairs, 2007).

For those patients with advancing dementia, Simard (2013) has described the significance of making connections through Namaste care. This involves a short period of sensory stimulation through the use of music, sounds and touch, colour, scents and food treats. All of these components are ways of connecting and communicating with a person for whom speech has limited meaning (Nicol and Nyatanga, 2017).

Interprofessional Communication Skills

Paramedics are expected to work effectively and professionally with other colleagues and agencies. This requirement is partly driven by the concept that 'two heads are better than one' but also that the experience and knowledge of others can enrich your own contribution. However, it is important to ensure that the patient is fully involved with this process (Moss, 2017).

At end of life, there may be a lack of awareness of which other agencies/colleagues may be able to positively contribute to difficulties or dilemmas. One way to address this may be to collate useful out-of-hours contact numbers for key professionals that you may need to contact, including the Macmillan nurses, palliative care team, district nurses and local oncology ward/unit involved in the patient's care. Sometimes it can take time to arrange community visits from the right people: in these circumstances it may be preferable to hand over concerns to the patient's GP or, if out of hours, advise the patient's relatives of a plan of action once key people are available to contact.

It is important to remember not to rush in; spend time reflecting on the best way forward. Be clear about your own role and understand the role of other agencies that you might call upon. Remember that interprofessional collaboration is the major factor in preventing tragedy from happening (Moss, 2017). Pooling the resources of a variety of professional staff will positively contribute to the holistic care of patients and their families.

Breaking Bad News

Handling awkward situations is one of the key features of palliative care and breaking bad news can to some extent be anticipated and prepared for. Although the responsibility of sharing bad news regarding a diagnosis usually lays in the hands of specialists, all healthcare professionals are increasingly being involved in breaking bad news (Kinghorn et al., 2007). Bad news can be any information that negatively alters a person's belief about what will happen in the future (Buckman, 1984). However, there is a need to consider how to deliver bad news and there are various frameworks designed to assist healthcare professionals with this task. Baile et al.

(2000) propose a six-step approach known as the SPIKES framework, which involves an assessment of the patient's perception and permission to fill in any blanks with the giving of knowledge and information that is evidenced based. The six-step approach to the SPIKES protocol is as follows:

S – **S**etting up an interview

P – Assessing the patient's **p**erception

I – Obtaining the patient's **i**nvitation

K – Giving **k**nowledge and information to the patient

E – Addressing the patient's **e**motions with **e**mpathetic response

S – **S**trategy and **s**ummary.

(Baile et al., 2000)

Honest disclosure regarding a prognosis or treatment options enables informed decision making (Mueller, 2002). This is important, especially at the end of life when it is vital that patients and their families understand what the likely outcomes of their decisions might be. For example, if a patient does not have a DNACPR decision/order but are reaching the end of life following a recent palliative diagnosis, they may not realise that if their family dial 999 because they suddenly stop breathing, this could lead to a resuscitation attempt that may be futile.

Really, the key objective of breaking bad news is for the paramedic to gather the necessary information about the patient's history, assess the current situation and determine what actions could be taken. They then need to explain these options to the patient and their relatives, while providing support and developing a plan to move forwards. It may be the case that caregivers simply do not realise their loved ones have entered the dying phase. Physical symptoms, including altered respiratory rate and effort, loss of consciousness, persistent dry mouth, or facial gestures demonstrating the presence of pain, are all a part of what is expected at the end of life. However, some people may simply not know this. Truth-telling and detailed explanation of the dying process is what is needed at this point. Often, paramedics may be in the penultimate position of delivering this information, which can be perceived as very bad news indeed by all those involved.

Truth-Telling in Clinical Practice

Pre-hospital clinicians are confronted with a myriad of difficult situations during end of life emergency calls (Waldrop et al., 2015). Sometimes a paramedic will be required to discuss the benefits and disadvantages of treatment options, especially if any decision requires transferring a patient to hospital. If the patient has expressed a desire to die at home, this needs to be taken into consideration. Relatives and caregivers can panic when they are not sure what they are dealing with and, as a result of their fear, will call the emergency services for assistance. Paramedics will need to assess the situation on arrival to determine what the expected outcome will be, what the prognosis is and whether the patient would benefit from being admitted to hospital or if there is any opportunity for further collaboration and involvement of other community services, such as the palliative care team.

The choice of whether to transport a patient to hospital or not in situations where the family are intensely reactive can feel like crisis management. Paramedics do a marvellous job of performing multifocal assessments of emergency end of life calls, which involve understanding the patient status while quickly identifying the family dynamics, which can have a huge influence on decision making (Waldrop et al., 2015). Perhaps interestingly, as many as 50% of family members do not understand the patient's diagnosis and prognosis (Jacobowski et al., 2010).

There is no guarantee that any conversation will be simple or straightforward, some may indeed take practitioners into uncharted territory of complexity where sensitive communication is key (Moss, 2017). There are no cut and dried routes to successful communication, as each situation will be different. However, there are certain factors that will impact upon the creation of a trusting relationship between the professional and the patient, such as age, race, gender, class and simple chemistry (Moss, 2017). Ultimately, the focus should be to facilitate a peaceful death and prevent undignified and inappropriate resuscitation attempts.

Referrals, Documentation and Follow-Up

Hoare et al. (2018) state that hospital admission for patients at end of life, particularly those who die shortly after admission, can be viewed as avoidable failures. Ambulance clinicians play a critical role in deciding whether dying patients should be transferred to hospital or whether they need to be referred to another member of the multidisciplinary team if their immediate needs cannot be met, e.g. the hospice at home team. The Health and Care Professions Council (HCPC) (2018) state that all paramedics must keep accurate records, giving full and clear accounts of the care and treatment given to patients or referrals made to other services. So, where patients do require transfer or follow-up treatment, this must be communicated verbally to the patient and their family, as well as documented in the patient's health record.

Hope and Communication

With a palliative diagnosis, hope for a cure often changes to hope for a good death. However, for some people, when they lose hope of a cure this can lead to a state of despair (Kemp, 2007). Hope is a concept that has sparked much debate among philosophers, psychologists, and healthcare professionals. Nurturing hope is an essential part of palliative care and requires a multiprofessional approach (McIntyre and Chaplin, 2007).

Paramedics need to get a sense of what patients and their relatives are hoping for at the end of life. Hope in its simplest form may be perceived by some patients and relatives as effective management of physical symptoms. When considering how to facilitate hope in patients approaching end of life there are three themes to consider (McIntyre and Chaplin, 2007). The first theme relates to comfort. Fundamental to this is effective pain and symptom management. If a patient is distressed, their capacity for hope is arguably reduced (McIntyre and Chaplin, 2007). The second theme relates to attachment and emphasises the importance of caring, supportive relationships with family and healthcare professionals as a mechanism of reducing the fear of abandonment at the end of life (McIntyre and Chaplin, 2007). The third and perhaps most important theme is the feeling of worth. Worth is linked to having a sense of meaning and purpose for living. Where advancing disease can diminish physical functioning, hope may appear to be lost or given up (Hockley, 1993). Fostering hope in patients receiving palliative care at the end of life is an essential component to effective communication.

Patients can quite easily determine occasions when they are not being told the truth. This may make them feel patronised, but equally if information is given too bluntly or tactlessly, they may feel disheartened (Randall and Downie, 2006). If patients are made to feel there is nothing to hope for, that feeling of hopelessness may lead to depression, increasing their suffering. There is no doubt that what practitioners say and the information they give will directly influence what patients are able to hope for and the way they see their future (Randall and Downie, 2006). However, there is professional guidance that states that it would not be ethical to foster false hope by avoiding the truth or making promises that can't be kept. Perhaps the key is to give patients a truthful portrayal of the probabilities from which they can then generate their own hopes (Randall and Downie, 2006).

Conclusion

All healthcare professionals use a range of communication skills to support patient-centred care that is safe and effective. In doing so they must ensure that patients receive all the information they need in a language and manner that they understand, and that supports informed decision making (Nicol and Nyatanga, 2017).

However, it is clear that there are many barriers to the delivery of effective and useful communication when patients are dying. Clinicians struggle to find a balance between providing real and honest information while still nurturing hope. However, the goals of palliative and end of life care remain consistent, in that the patient's needs and desires about the death they wish to have must be met where possible.

To achieve this in practice, it is important for paramedics to examine their own feelings and apprehensions about death. They should also seek training and advice in communicating with patients approaching the end of life. This extra training should also include advance directives and management of family conflict.

To truly support the end of life decisions or wishes of patients, all healthcare professionals need to be prepared to deal with high-level emotions and, at times, unrealistic expectations from patients and their carers. To do this effectively consideration must be given to how information and advice can be conveyed without prejudice and in a timely and appropriate manner. Such an approach is achievable with some thought and anticipation of possible problems. To assist with this, here are four scenarios that will challenge clinicians to think about their approach.

Case Studies

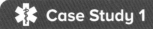 Case Study 1

Joseph is a widower with end-stage heart failure. He lives alone with daily visits from his daughter Jane. This morning Jane makes a call to 999 because her father's breathing has become increasingly laboured overnight, he is confused and agitated and she can't seem to communicate with him. Jane tells the call handler that Joseph has a DNACPR form at home but that she feels useless, doesn't know what to do and needs help.

When you arrive at the property it is clear that Joseph is now experiencing Cheyne-Stokes breathing. Jane is panicking and doesn't seem to understand what is happening.

- How would you break the bad news to Jane that Joseph has entered the dying process?
- Who else could you contact to support Jane and her father?

Case Study 2

Sima is a 60-year-old woman with strong family values. She was diagnosed with terminal lung cancer three weeks ago and given three months to live. Sima lives at home with her husband and youngest daughter Alicia. This evening at 20.00, Sima started to cough uncontrollably; as she was not able to stop coughing, Alicia dialled 999. Alicia advises the call handler that Sima is now coughing up bright red blood and is becoming increasingly distressed. Alicia advises the call handler that Sima wants to go to hospital.

When you arrive at the property, Sima has had a small amount of haemoptysis. She does have bilateral crepitations on auscultation but her saturations are 94%. You ask to see her care plan and you are given some notes from the palliative care team that have been visiting Sima at home. You note that ventolin is prescribed and you ask the family if Sima has used her inhaler. The family say that they don't understand what an inhaler is and give you a bag of medications. It would seem that Sima has not been taking anything to manage her symptoms.

- Reflecting on the case study and considering the fundamental aspects of communication, how would you as the attending paramedic manage this situation?
- Who else could you contact to help support Sima and her family with her end of life care plan, taking into consideration that it is now past 20.00?

✥ Case Study 3

Vivian is a 53-year-old woman who had a left-sided CVA two years ago. She recovered quite well initially but six weeks ago had an extension of her stroke, which has left her with a left-sided hemiparesis and loss of speech. She has been moved to a nursing home as she had no rehabilitation potential and required too much care to return home. The nursing home have dialled 999 this morning as Vivian has become increasingly distressed overnight and started frothing at the mouth. They are concerned she may have further extended her CVA.

On your arrival it appears clear that Vivian has had recurrent seizures. There is some evidence of blood-stained sputum around her mouth where she appears to have bitten her tongue. The nursing home staff show you a DNACPR form that was completed four days previously by the consultant managing her care. Vivian is now settled with a GCS score of 9 but the staff are keen to get her transferred to hospital and they have packed her overnight bag and medications.

When you arrive at the home the nursing home staff refuse to keep Vivian and insist you transport her to hospital, despite a valid DNACPR form and an expectation that survival is not expected.

- How would you communicate with the staff and manage their expectations in a supportive and appropriate way?

✥ Case Study 4

Paolo is a 70-year-old man who has Stage 4 bowel cancer with liver and lung metastases. He lives at home with his wife Joan, who is a retired nurse. Paolo has been managing his pain quite well with morphine patches and Oramorph as required. Overnight though, his pain has increased twofold and he has been crying out in agony. Joan has dialled 999 as the GP surgery is closed and she does not know what else she can give Paolo for the pain.

When you arrive to assess Paolo he is visibly distressed. You are able to gain IV access and give him some IV paracetamol, which helps only a little. Paolo is very keen to remain at home but his wife is worried that when you leave, he will not be able to cope with the pain.

- Who can you contact at the weekend to assist with pain management?
- Is there anything else you could do or suggest to help Paolo keep his wish of remaining at home?

References

Ali M (2017). Communication Skills 2: Overcoming the barriers to effective communication. *Nursing Times*, 114(1): 40–42.

Baile WF et al. (2000). SPIKES – A six-step protocol for delivering bad news: application to the patient with cancer. *Oncologist*, 5: 302–311.

Bateman N (1995). *Advocacy Skills: A Handbook for Human Service Professionals.* Aldershot: Ashgate Arena.

Buckman R (1984). Breaking bad news: why is it still so difficult? *BMJ*, 288(6430): 1597–1599.

Coulter A and Collins AB (2011). *Making Shared Decision-Making a Reality: No Decisions About Me Without Me.* London: The King's Fund.

Davenport D (2013). The basics of clinical supervision. *Nursing in Practice.* Available at: https://www.nursinginpractice.com/article/basics-clinical-supervision.

Department for Constitutional Affairs (2007). *Mental Capacity Act 2005: Code of Practice.* London: The Stationery Office.

Ebell M, Becker LA and Barry HC (1998). Survival after in-hospital cardiopulmonary resuscitation. *Journal of General Internal Medicine*, 13(12): 805–816.

Ewer M, Kish S and Martin C (2001). Characteristics of cardiac arrest in cancer patients as a predictor of survival after cardiopulmonary resuscitation. *Cancer*, 92(7): 1905–1912.

Farrer, K (2007). Pain control. In Kinghorn S and Gaines S (eds). *Palliative Nursing, Improving End-of-Life Care.* London: Balliere Tindall Elsevier, 23–41.

General Medical Council (2010). *Treatment and care towards the end of life: good practice in decision making.* Available at: https://www.gmc-uk.org/-/media/documents/Treatment_and_care_towards_the_end_of_life___English_1015.pdf_48902105.pdf.

Health and Care Professions Council (2018). *Standards of Conduct, Performance and Ethics.* Available at: http://www.hpc-uk.org/standards/standards-of-conduct-performance-and-ethics/.

Health Education England (2017). *End of Life Care Core Skills Education and Training Framework.* Available at: https://www.eolc.co.uk/educational/end-of-life-care-core-skills-education-and-training-framework/#.

Higgins D (2010). Care of the dying patient: a guide for nurses. In Jevon P et al. (eds), *Care of the Dying and Deceased Patient.* Chichester: Wiley-Blackwell: 1–36.

Hoare S, Kelly MP and Prothero L (2018). Ambulance staff and end-of-life hospital admissions: a qualitative interview study. *Palliative Medicine*, 32(9): 1465–1473.

Hockley J (1993). The concept of hope and the will to live. *Palliative Medicine*, 7: 181–186.

Jacobowski NL et al. (2010). Communication in critical care: family rounds in the intensive care unit. *American Journal of Critical Care*, 19(5): 421–430.

Kemp C (2007). Spiritual care across cultures. In Kuebler KK et al. (eds), *Palliative Practices: An Interdisciplinary Approach.* St. Louis: Elsevier Mosby.

Kinghorn S, Gaines S and Satterley G (2007). Communication in advanced illness: challenges and opportunities. In Kinghorn S and Gaines S (eds), *Palliative Nursing, Improving End-of-Life Care.* London: Balliere Tindall Elsevier: 95–125.

Kozlowska L and Doboszynska A (2012). Nurses' nonverbal methods of communication with patients in the terminal phase. *International Journal of Palliative Nursing*, 18(1): 40–46.

Kuebler KK, Heidrich DE and Esper P (2007). *End-of-life Care: Clinical Practice Guidelines* (2nd ed.). Milton Keynes: Saunders Elsevier.

Maguire P et al., (1996). Helping cancer patients disclose their concerns. *European Journal of Cancer*, 32: 78–81.

Marie Curie (2019). *Communication Difficulties*. Available at: https://www.mariecurie.org.uk/professionals/palliative-care-knowledge-zone/individual-needs/communication-difficulties.

McIntyre R and Chaplin J (2007). Facilitating hope in palliative care. In Kinghorn S and Gaines S (eds), *Palliative Nursing, Improving End-of-Life Care*. London: Balliere Tindall Elsevier, 111–128.

Miller S and Dorman S (2014). Resuscitation decisions for patients dying in the community: a qualitative interview study of general practitioner perspectives. *Palliative Medicine*, 28(8): 1053–1061.

Moore CD (2005). Advance care planning. In Kuebler KK et al. (eds), *Palliative Practices: An Interdisciplinary Approach*. St. Louis: Elsevier Mosby.

Moss B (2017). *Communication Skills in Health and Social Care* (4th ed.). London: SAGE.

Mueller PS (2002). Breaking bad news to patients: the spikes approach can make this difficult task easier. *Postgraduate Medicine*, 112(3): 15–18.

National Cancer Institute (2017). *NCI Dictionary of Cancer Terms*. Available at: https://www.cancer.gov/publications/dictionaries/cancer-terms

National Institute for Health and Care Excellence (2004). *Improving Supportive and Palliative Care for Adults with Cancer*. Available at: http://www.nice.org.uk/guidance/csg4.

Nicol J and Nyatanga B (2017). *Palliative and End of Life Care in Nursing* (2nd ed.). London: Sage.

Penrod J et al. (2011). End-of-life caregiving trajectories. *Clinical Nursing Research*. 20(1): 7–24.

Randall F and Downie RS (2006). *The Philosophy of Palliative Care: Critique and Reconstruction*. Oxford: Oxford University Press.

ReSPECT (2017). *Recommended Summary Plan for Emergency Care and Treatment*. Available at: http://www.respectprocess.org.uk.

Richardson M (2018). *Advanced Communication Skills*. London: Matthew Richardson.

Rodenbach RA et al. (2016). Relationships between personal attitudes about death and communication with terminally ill patients: how oncology clinicians grapple with mortality. *Patient Education and Counselling*, 99: 356–363.

Simard J (2013). *The End of Life Namaste Care Program for People with Dementia*. Baltimore: Health Professions Press.

Trevithick P (2012). *Social Work Skills: A Practice Handbook* (3rd ed.). Maidenhead: Open University Press.

Waldrop DP et al. (2015). 'We are strangers walking into their life-changing event': How pre-hospital providers manage emergency calls at the end of life. *American Academy of Hospice and Palliative Medicine*, 50(3): 328–334.

Webb L (2011). Introduction to communication skills. In: Webb L (eds), *Nursing Communication Skills in Practice*. Oxford: University Press: 3–17.

Wiese CH et al. (2009). Quality of out of hospital palliative emergency care depends on the expertise of the emergency medical team – a prospective multi-centre analysis. *Support Care Cancer*, 17: 1499–1506.

Wittenberg-Lyles E et al. (2013). *Communication in Palliative Nursing*. New York: Oxford University Press.

Chapter 6

Care of the Dying Patient

Tania Blackmore

Introduction

For most people, home is their preferred place of death and where they want to be cared for in the dying phase of their illness (Hoare et al., 2018), and because of this, national healthcare policy is trying to facilitate this preference. According to the literature there is not much data on the frequency of paramedic attendance to patients at end of life, but a recent study in the West Midlands has suggested that palliative and end of life care makes up a substantial part of a paramedic's practice. With 33% of paramedics in the study reporting that they get calls to palliative patients on average once a shift and a further 29% stating that they see palliative patients between every two to five shifts in their practice (Munday, 2010, cited in Pettifer and Bronnert, 2013). These attendances to patients are usually in response to anxious loved ones and relatives dialling 999 as a reaction to a rapid deterioration of the dying patient at end of life (Pettifer and Bronnert, 2013). In the past the ambulance service was seen as a transportation service, but now the role of the paramedic has extended and paramedics have to treat a whole plethora of complex needs of patients within the home environment (Kirk et al., 2017). In a study looking at paramedics and their perceptions of their confidence in caring for patients at end of life, 78% of paramedics agreed that caring for end of life patients is a key part of their practice, but worryingly 51% of those paramedics reported their end of life training as poor (Kirk et al., 2017).

This chapter will explore the essential requirements needed in care of the dying patient in order to assist the paramedic to develop their skills in end of life care, they are as follows:

- Ten key elements for care of the dying patient
- Recognising death
- Anticipatory medication
- Symptom control at end of life
- The doctrine of double effect
- Do Not Attempt Cardiopulmonary Resuscitation orders (DNACPR)

- What is a good death?

- Care after death

- Bereavement, grief and loss

- Do our personal beliefs affect our clinical practice?

Ten Key Elements for Care of the Dying Patient

It has been suggested that we need a radical change in health systems to enable clinicians such as paramedics to care for dying patients at home with adequate support in the best interest of patients at end of life (Ellershaw and Lakhani, 2013). International and UK research has identified ten key elements that are necessary for achieving the best care for dying patients; these elements also appear in the General Medical Council and NICE guidance on caring for patients in the dying phase (Ellershaw and Lakhani, 2013). These key elements are as follows:

1. Recognition that the patient is dying.

2. Communication with the patient (if possible) and always with family and loved ones.

3. Spiritual care (consideration of the dying patient's beliefs and rituals).

4. Anticipatory medication.

5. Review of the necessary clinical interventions (this could be the stopping of unnecessary drugs and clinical observations).

6. Hydration review (including an explanation to the carers/loved ones and relatives of the cessation of artificial hydration).

7. Nutritional review (including an explanation to the carers/loved ones and relatives of the cessation of nutrition).

8. Full discussion of the plan of care with the patient (if possible) and/or carer/relatives/loved ones.

9. Regular assessment of the patient (holistic symptom control – physically, psychologically, spiritually and socially).

10. Maintained dignified care of the patient after death.

(Adapted from Ellershaw and Lakhani, 2013)

Recognising Death

As discussed in Chapter 2 – Defining Palliative Care, one of the main criticisms of the Liverpool Care Pathway Review (Department of Health, 2013) was the inability of clinicians to recognise and acknowledge the dying process. The symptoms seen in the dying phase have been summarise by van der Werff et al. (2012) in a conceptual model of the signs and symptoms of the dying phase (see Figure 6.1).

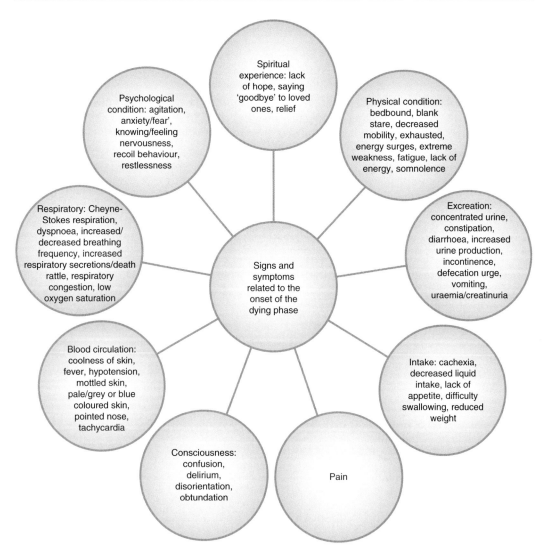

Figure 6.1 Conceptual model of the signs and symptoms of the dying phase
Source: Adapted from van der Werff et al, 2012

Since this review was conducted, research has attempted to better define the dying process with a systematic review looking at the biomarkers of dying cancer patients in a bid to give clear clinical definitions of physiological changes that happen as part of the dying process (Reid et al., 2017). The review concluded that the dying process involved biomarker changes in four different biological areas:

1. **Systematic and haematological changes** – with elevated inflammatory markers.

2. **Cancer anorexia** – cachexia syndrome defined by poor prealbumin levels.

3. **Hepatic dysfunction** – indicating a poor prognosis.

4. **Electrolyte changes** – the most common aetiology being inappropriate secretion of antidiuretic hormone.

However, the review doubted the use of these markers to help as prognostic tools in dying patients in frontline clinical practice (Reid et al., 2017). If we look at the diagram (van der Werff et al., 2012) we can see how the biological changes would contribute to the symptoms seen in the dying phase. In addition, please look at the JRCALC Clinical Guidelines (2019: 56) – 'Signs that a patient is at the very end of life'.

To summarise, onset of the dying phase usually manifests in the following way:

- **Changes in breathing patterns** – both reduced respiratory rate, rapid breathing, noisy breathing, sighing

- **Paleness of the skin** – may look mottled, blue tinged, cool to touch

- **Increased drowsiness** – sleeping most of the time

- **Confusion** – disorientated in time, place and person

- **Decreased urine output** – concentrated or very little output

- **Reduced oral intake** – refusing food and fluid, unable to swallow

- **Pinched nose** – in palliative care, clinicians often notice a pointed nose

- **Reduced communication** – letting go of social connections, lack of eye contact

- **Fear** – some patients may become anxious

- **Saying goodbye** – patient has an awareness that they are dying and expresses this to their family and loved ones

- **Seeking permission from loved ones to go** – patients ask if it's OK to stop fighting and not to carry on

- A **gradual shutting down** of all functions, physical, emotional and social.

It's important for paramedics to note the signs discussed identify the way that the majority of people die who die from an expected death due to a known illness or old age with no dramatic occurrences or medical emergencies. This is just a gradual shutting down of all the body's physiological systems and an emotional and social withdrawal from their family and loved ones. This dying process is common at the end stage of all diseases. Patterns of disease are changing and because treatment options are improving, people are living longer with chronic illness. Chronic illnesses, such as ischaemic heart disease, cerebrovascular disease and chronic obstructive pulmonary disease will be the most common diseases diagnosed in the world by 2020 (Wallerstedt et al., 2012). The number of deaths worldwide is set to change from 57 million in 2015 to 70 million in the next 15 years because of ageing populations (Bone et al., 2018). For the latest guidance on the end stage of any specific chronic illness, please refer to the National Institute for Health and Care Excellence (NICE) guidelines (2020).

Anticipatory Medication

The Royal College of Physicians (RCP) 2016 end of life audit studied 9302 deaths in 142 trusts in England. They noted the most common symptoms of death and the percentages of deaths in which these symptoms were controlled: (1) pain – 79% controlled; (2) agitation/delirium – 72% controlled; (3) breathing difficulties – 68% controlled; (4) noisy breathing/death rattle – 62% controlled; (5) nausea/vomiting – 55% controlled. What is of note is that there is the clinical ability to manage all these symptoms at end of life successfully with consideration of the four most common symptoms seen and evidenced in the literature.

Prescribing within the four common symptom groups of end of life care is known as anticipatory prescribing and consists of the following four groups of drugs – analgesics, anti-secretory, antiemetic and anxiolytic/sedatives. It is well acknowledged in the literature that unfortunately the majority of dying patients in European countries do not receive the necessary drugs to relieve their symptoms at end of life (Lindqvist et al., 2013). A study of the four essential drugs needed to provide quality care was conducted in nine European countries, including the UK. One hundred and thirty-five palliative care clinicians took part (Lindqvist et al., 2013). The results of the study concluded that out of a total of thirty-five anticipatory drugs identified, the most common drug choices were as follows:

- For **anxiety**: midazolam and lorazepam
- For **dyspnoea/breathlessness**: morphine
- For **nausea and vomiting**: metoclopramide and haloperidol
- For **pain**: morphine
- For **respiratory secretions**: hyoscine (reported as hyoscine, hyoscine hydrobromide, or hyoscine butyl bromide and glycopyrronium)
- For **terminal restlessness and agitation**: midazolam and haloperidol.

(Lindqvist et al., 2013)

Pain at End of Life

Pain is often seen in dying patients and research shows it is often not managed well, especially in non-cancer dying patients. It is a very unpleasant and sensory experience that directly impacts adversely on the emotions of patients (Steindal et al., 2011). It is important to consider the dying patient's total pain, which encompasses not only the physical cause of pain but the psychological, social and spiritual aspects of pain (Albert, 2017). What is of note, and reassuring for those paramedics that administer opioids to dying patients, is that there is no evidence that administering opioid analgesia in advanced diseases shortens patient's lives or reduces survival; in fact there is evidence available that uncontrolled cancer pain has a correlation with shorter survival rates (Thompson, 2018).

The majority of palliative patients will be able to take their analgesia by mouth but as the patient enters the dying phase this is often not possible, and the subcutaneous route of analgesia administration is used. The first line of administration in the subcutaneous route of opioid analgesia for the end of life patient is morphine. The initial dose will be based on the amount the patient has been taking orally, but if they are opioid naïve (meaning they are not currently on any opioid medication), the initial dose would be 2.5 mg to 5 mg subcutaneously (SC), when necessary – pro re nata (PRN), 2–4 hourly (Dickman, 2012). The frequency is often 1–2 hourly in specialist palliative care units or on palliative prescriptions.

Patients who are not opioid naïve and have already been on regular oral opioids but are now unable to swallow can have their oral dose converted to a continuous subcutaneous infusion (CSCI), also known as a syringe driver. A point in practice is that patients who have been on long-term codeine, either as codeine by itself or in combination with paracetamol as co-codamol, are often seen as opiate naïve and this is not the case. Codeine is an opioid analgesia and is ten times less potent than morphine (Dickman and Schneider, 2016).

The Conversion of Oral Opioids to Subcutaneous Opioids

Oral Morphine to Subcutaneous Morphine – 2:1 Conversion

Divide the total daily 24-hour dose by 2 to give the total that should be administered over 24 hours via the syringe driver. So if the patient's total oral intake of morphine over 24 hours was 80 mg, then 40 mg of morphine would be put in the syringe driver (adapted from Dickman, 2012: 54).

Oral Morphine to Subcutaneous Diamorphine – 3:1 Conversion

Divide the total daily 24-hour dose by 3 to give the total that should be administered over 24 hours via the syringe driver. So if the patient's total oral intake of morphine over 24 hours was 90 mg of morphine, then 30 mg of diamorphine would be put in the syringe driver (adapted from Dickman, 2012: 54).

Oral Oxycodone to Subcutaneous Oxycodone – 1.5:1 Conversion

Divide the total daily 24-hour dose by 1.5 to give the total that should be administered over 24 hours via the syringe driver. So if the patient's total oral intake of oxycodone over 24 hours was 90 mg, then 60 mg of oxycodone would be put in the syringe driver (adapted from Dickman, 2012: 54).

Oral Morphine to Subcutaneous Alfentanil – 30:1 Conversion

Divide the total 24-hour dose by 30 to give the total dose to be administered over 24 hours via a syringe driver. So if the patient's oral dose of morphine is 60 mg, then 2 mg of alfentanil will be put into the syringe driver. Alfentanil is often used in general anaesthesia and it is particularly useful at end of life as an analgesia for patients with renal failure (Dickman and Schneider, 2016). Alfentanil has a rapid onset of action so is effective within 5 minutes and lasts about 1 hour. It is useful in end of life care (Dickman and Schneider, 2016; Lindqvist et al., 2013), but because of its rapid onset and short action it is best administered over 24 hours via a syringe driver.

NB For further information on syringe driver administration, such as rates and diluents, please look at *The Syringe Driver – Continuous Subcutaneous Infusions in Palliative Care* (Dickman and Schneider, 2016). See also the conversion chart in Chapter 4 of this textbook (page 79).

Key Points

- End of life patients often need analgesia for severe to moderate pain.

- Many palliative care clinicians believe there is a failing to address the pain and suffering of terminally ill patients, which violates the ethical principles of beneficence and non-maleficence.

- Paramedics have a duty of care, underpinned by their professional registration, to care for dying patients to the best of their competency (Parkinson, 2015; JRCALC, 2019).

Nausea at End of Life

Nausea and vomiting are common symptoms in the dying patient, and are caused by multiple receptor pathways both in the brain and in the gastrointestinal tract itself (Albert, 2017). Antiemetics that focus on the dopaminergic pathways, such as metoclopramide, prochlorperazine and haloperidol, are often the first-line medications used for nausea and vomiting as inhibitors of the brain's chemoreceptor trigger zone receptors (Bayatrizi, 2014; Hodgkinson et al., 2016; Ruijs et al., 2013). In paramedic practice, ondansetron is often used as the first-line medication for nausea and vomiting. The use of ondansetron in end of life patients is underpinned in the research, with studies showing that the use of ondansetron is often far more effective than the older dopaminergic medications, such as metoclopramide (Albert, 2017).

The choice of antiemetic for patients at end of life should ideally be based on what mechanism is causing the symptom and whether the nausea and vomiting is reversible, the side effect of the antiemetic to be used – which may be increased sedation as a benefit of using that particular antiemetic – and the compatibility of the chosen antiemetic with other medication the dying patient is receiving (Hodgkinson et al., 2016) (refer to Chapter 4 – Symptom Management, for further guidance).

One of the reversible causes of nausea and vomiting in end of life patients is constipation (Albert, 2017). This is of note because if a palliative patient's constipation is managed earlier in the disease trajectory, this can improve symptoms such as nausea and pain when the patient deteriorates as part of the dying phase. Although choice of first-line antiemetic varies from health sector to health sector, there is a consensus that if an antiemetic is required, the best practice is to give it as a CSCI rather than a PRN medication so that the dying patient's nausea and vomiting is controlled resulting in overall better symptom control (Rayment and Ward, 2011) (see Chapter 4 – Symptom Management, for more information about nausea and vomiting).

Antiemetic Drugs at End of Life

- **Metoclopramide** – 10–20 mg, 6–8 hourly, orally or 10 mg SC (Albert, 2017).

- **Haloperidol** – Stat dose 1.5–3 mg SC or over 24 hours 1.5–20 mg via a CSCI (Rayment and Ward, 2011).

- **Cyclizine** – Stat dose 25–50 mg SC or over 24 hours 100–150 mg via a CSCI. Please note incompatible with hyoscine butyl bromide (Rayment and Ward, 2011). It is also important to know that cyclizine can exacerbate congestive heart failure, so must be avoided in patients with this condition (Dickman, 2012).

- **Levomepromazine** – Usually the choice of antiemetic if no identifiable cause can be found for the dying patient's nausea and vomiting (Dickman, 2012). Stat dose 6.25–12.5 mg or the most efficient way at end of life via a CSCI 6.25–25 mg (Rayment and Ward, 2011).

- **Ondansetron** – Stat dose 4–8 mg BD or 8–16 mg via a CSCI (Dickman and Schneider, 2016). A 5-HT$_3$ antagonist, a good option if the nausea is caused by renal failure, recent chemotherapy, bowel obstruction or gastric cancers (Dickman, 2012).

Delirium and Agitation at End of Life

Patients in the dying phase are often delirious, agitated and restless and this is not only distressing for the dying patient themselves but for their loved ones and family. A literature review of end of life symptoms suggests that the frequency of delirium in palliative patients is 62%, increasing to 88% in those patients in the days and hours before death, and it is said to be the most distressing psychological symptom, but it is often not addressed by clinicians and frequently undertreated (Finucane et al., 2017). The symptoms of delirium, as discussed in Chapter 4 – Symptom Management, are restlessness, agitation, hallucinations, delusions, abnormal thought processes, lethargy and increased activity – both hyperactive and hypoactive symptoms may be noted (Lawley and Hewison, 2017). The causes of delirium and agitation should always be assessed, considered and treated, if possible, at end of life.

Possible causes:

- Alcohol/nicotine withdrawal
- Biochemical disturbances, such as hypercalcaemia or hypoglycaemia
- Brain tumours/metastases
- Constipation
- Adverse drug reactions
- Infection
- Pain.

(Dickman, 2012)

The literature available on the treatment of delirium in end of life patients highlights that there is limited evidence to support specific uses of certain medication and that there is a great need for further investigation into the pathophysiology of delirium (Lawley and Hewison, 2017). The current drugs used in delirium will be discussed here with reference to Dickman (2012). Delirium and agitation and their mechanisms are discussed in greater depth in Chapter 4 – Symptom Management.

Drugs Used for Delirium at End of Life

- **Haloperidol** – 0.5–2.5 mg PRN subcutaneously. If more than two doses are required in a 24-hour period, consider commencing a CSCI, with a starting dose of 2.5 mg of haloperidol over 24 hours (Dickman, 2012).

Drugs Used for Agitation at End of Life

- **Midazolam** – 2.5–5 mg PRN subcutaneously. If more than two doses are required in a 24-hour period, consider commencing a CSCI, with a minimum of 10 mg of midazolam over 24 hours (Dickman and Schneider, 2016).

Respiratory Secretions and Dyspnoea at End of Life

It is common in dying patients that their breathing is noisy and that they produce respiratory secretions: the noisy breathing is sometimes described as the 'death rattle'. There are also changes in the pattern of breathing, with long gaps between breaths – apnoea. This abnormal pattern of breathing is also described as Cheyne-Stokes respiration, which is characterised by deep breathing that is sometimes faster (hyperpnoea) or alternates between temporarily stopping (apnoea) and hyperpnoea. It is thought that the patient is usually not aware of their noisy and changing breathing, but this pattern of changed breathing is very distressing for relatives and loved ones of the dying patient to witness (Albert, 2017). The symptoms of dying are low oxygen saturation, death rattle, Cheyne-Stokes respiration and both an increase and decrease in respiratory rate (van der Werff et al., 2012). Relatives and loved ones should be advised and reassured that this is a normal part of the dying process and does not indicate that the dying patient is distressed, uncomfortable or in pain.

Anticholinergic drugs are prescribed as part of the anticipatory drugs in end of life care, but it must be noted that there is sparse evidence of high quality data to support their effectiveness in controlling respiratory secretions and aiding breathing at end of life (Albert, 2017). Key to optimising the effectiveness of these drugs is to initiate their use as soon as the 'death rattle' or noisy breathing occurs (Dickman and Schneider, 2016). It is imperative to understand that the non-pharmacological measures in symptom control of respiratory secretions and dyspnoea are more important than the pharmacological. Emphasis of care for these symptoms should be aimed at reassurance of the dying patient and their relatives and loved ones. Simple measures, such as repositioning the patient, perhaps propping them up with extra pillows and constant verbal reassurance, can ease symptoms (see Chapter 4 – Symptom Management). The available drugs are stated below.

Drugs Used for Respiratory Secretions at End of Life

- **Glycopyrronium** – 0.2 mg subcutaneously PRN as prescribed or 0.6–1.2 mg via a CSCI over 24 hours (Dickman, 2012; Dickman and Schneider, 2016).

- **Hyoscine butyl bromide** – 20 mg subcutaneously PRN as prescribed or 60–180 mg via a CSCI over 24 hours (Dickman, 2012; Dickman and Schneider, 2016).

- **Hyoscine hydrobromide** – 0.4 mg subcutaneously as prescribed or 1.2–2.4 mg via a CSCI over 24 hours (Dickman, 2012; Dickman and Schneider, 2016; Lindqvist et al., 2013).

As described in Chapter 4 – Symptom Management, breathlessness or dyspnoea is often part of the panic cycle and as such it is advised that non-pharmacological measures such as fan therapy, moving air across the face and verbal reassurance can diminish symptoms. If pharmacological treatment is needed, midazolam 2.5–5 mg PRN can be used or added to the CSCI over 24 hours (Dickman, 2012). Opiates such as morphine are often used at end of life to alleviate the symptoms of breathlessness. Please note that when opiates are used at the appropriate doses they do not supress the respiratory system and do not hasten death but help to reduce the distressing symptom of air hunger (Albert, 2017). Consider putting morphine into the CSCI over 24 hours if effective for dyspnoea (Dickman, 2012).

The Doctrine of Double Effect

The use of high dose opiates, sedative and antiemetics in end of life care causes much anxiety in paramedic practice because of the known side effects of respiratory depression and the thought that these drugs not only help symptom control in the dying patient but the fear that they may also hasten death. This theory is discussed as the principle of 'double effect' and is rooted in Christian philosophy and the teachings and writing of Saint Thomas Aquinas (1225–1274). He suggested that one act can have two effects, one being an intended good act and the other being an unintended bad act. The doctrine of double effect is said to have little place in current end of life practice, as when drugs are prescribed correctly in end of life care they do not hasten death as they are titrated to the individual patient and there is never a reason to give a lethal dose of drugs to a patient to control suffering (Regnard et al., 2011). Further evidence of a recent systematic review of the literature of the doctrine of double effect confirmed the theory has little relevance in palliative care because appropriate clinical prescribing does not cause death (Gannon, 2019). The paramedic can be reassured in practice by the evidence that the use of end of life medication in clinical practice is solely for symptomatic relief of the patient, not to hasten death, and a knowledge of the research can help relieve the anxiety surrounding the administration of those drugs.

Do Not Attempt Cardiopulmonary Resuscitation Order (DNACPR)

End of life care patients, whose preferred place of care is home, should have a DNACPR order in their home, care home or nursing home. This is completed by the most senior clinician in charge of their care, which can be the consultant in the acute sector, their general practitioner or a clinical nurse specialist from the hospice. Ideally a copy of the DNACPR should be shared with the ambulance service, GP and all teams involved in the care of the patient. It is good practice that the order is discussed in advance with the patient's family and caregivers and that they agree with it (Collis and Al-Qurainy, 2013). Reassurance should be given to the patient, loved ones and family that a DNACPR is not an indication that the patient will receive no care or symptom control, but is just a means to indicate that resuscitation would be futile and not effective (Collis and Al-Qurainy, 2013).

A recent UK study explored paramedic attitudes towards DNACPR (Armitage and Jones, 2017) and four themes emerged: (1) communication – that communication is needed that paramedic crews can access before attending patients, and that even when a DNAR is in place this is not always available; (2) education – more training is needed for paramedics in the legal requirements and how to educate and pass information to patients, family and carers; (3) responsibilities – whose responsibility was it to discuss DNARs with the patient, carers, and family? What if the form is not completed properly? What about review dates? (4) patient's wishes – were the patient's wishes documented as part of the DNAR process? Further research underpins concerns around documentation and communication with family and caregivers when paramedics treat patients with DNAR, with 70% reporting validity of documentation, fear of conflict with family, 50%, and fear of litigation, 46%, as concerns (Kirk et al., 2017). When looking at the literature on how paramedics view DNARs and caring for end of life patients, the recurring theme is reports of lack of training, education and knowledge when dealing with this group of patients (Armitage and Jones, 2017; Kirk et al., 2017; Pettifer and Bronnert, 2013).

What is a Good Death?

It can be hard to define what constitutes a good death, as the factors are different for each individual patient at end of life, but the research literature does agree on recurring general themes, which emphasise the need for a holistic approach in care of the dying patient. Such an approach should encompass not only the physical symptom-control needs of the patient in the dying phase, as discussed in anticipatory medication provisions, but also acknowledge the social, psychological and emotional needs of the patient at end of life.

These components were confirmed in a recent UK literature review, which concluded the following factors associated with achieving a good death:

- Pain and symptom management
- Clear decision making
- Preparation for death
- Life completion
- Contributing to others
- Affirmation of the whole person.

(Read and Macbride-Stewart, 2018)

The essential social, emotional and psychological factors that contribute to achieving a good death for our patients are as follows: the patient maintains social engagement and relationships, and has empathetic and proactive carers, who are confident, have ability, death awareness and are not only able to support the dying patient but also are able to support the family and loved ones after the death (Holdsworth, 2015; Kastbom et al., 2017). Looking at both Meier et al., (2016) and Holdsworth (2015), the consensus is that one of the key elements of attaining a good death for our patients is achieving preferences in place of care, which is obviously a poignant aspect in paramedic practice when relatives call 999 as the patient deteriorates at end of life and paramedics have to make clinical decisions on whether to treat the patient at home or transport to the hospital. The research underlines three components stated by end of life patients as essential in their perception of achieving a good death: (1) not to be a burden to the family; (2) the presence of family; (3) the resolution of unfinished business (Yun et al., 2018).

Therefore, achieving a good death for end of life patients is care not only of the dying patient but also their loved ones; the loved ones are forced into the role of decision makers in the care of the dying patient and this makes communication with family complex in the dying phase (Waldrop et al., 2018). Family members of a dying patient often call the ambulance service because of the overwhelming anxiety and distress they are facing as they watch their dying loved one deteriorate and enter the actively dying phase at the end of the disease trajectory. The paramedic and all clinicians that care for patients at end of life have to have great empathy and employ methods of intense and continuous communication with not only the dying patient but their loved ones and relatives (Galiana et al., 2019). This dying phase often presents clinicians with a situation that they cannot control, which is incredibly stressful not only to the patient but for loved ones and family members (Galiana et al., 2019). When considering what is a good death, it is essential that the discussion incorporates the experiences of the patient's loved ones and families, as these people are those who have to live on with the memory of the death; a good death is not just the dying process or the moment of death but also the time immediately after death (Holdsworth, 2015). These factors are very important to remember in the context of paramedic practice; when you are rushed, and the patient has died, there is still the family to be considered and care for before you sign off for your next call. There is a plethora of research that concludes that there is a link between the relative's feelings about the manner of their loved one's death and how they go on to grieve (Wilson et al., 2016).

Care After Death

Care after the death is extremely important. As discussed above, the deceased patient must be treated in a way that is congruent with the cultural, spiritual and psychosocial wishes of their loved ones (Olausson and Ferrell, 2013). For specific paramedic guidance in clinical procedure please refer to the JRCALC guidelines on 'Care after Death' (2019: 56). Do not presume that as you the paramedic know that the patient has died, the patient's family and loved ones are also aware of the death, especially if the patient has died during your visit.

Do the following:

1. Use direct language, i.e. dead or died.

2. Allow the family and loved ones to express their grief, i.e. don't try to supress emotional outbursts of the family/loved ones because you feel uncomfortable.

3. You can say you are sorry for their loss.

4. Ask them if they have any questions.

5. If you are unsure of any aspects around the death, such as informing the coroners, GP or hospice of an expected death of a known palliative patient with a DNAR, seek advice from the on-call GP service, ambulance control or phone the local hospice for advice.

6. Ask the family about any religious preferences/procedures after death that are important to their beliefs, i.e. in some forms of Buddhism it is sometimes not allowed to touch the body immediately after death as this is seen as hindering reincarnation.

7. There is never a reason to rush your call out; this time is precious and it's vital to get it right for the family.

8. Signpost the family to further support, such as the hospice, funeral directors, on-call GP.

Informing loved ones that a patient has died is extremely difficult and even the most experienced clinicians find it hard. Breaking bad news as a paramedic never gets easier, but you get better at doing it. In truth if it ever gets easy to deliver the news that someone has died or is dying then this should be examined. Perhaps that seems too direct, but we should always feel some emotion to tragedy and if we don't, this is a red flag that as a clinician we may need some professional psychological support (see also Chapter 5 – Enhanced Communication Skills for information on breaking bad news).

Bereavement, Grief and Loss

When discussing end of life care, it is essential to look at the concepts of loss, grief and bereavement to understand the social connections that occur with families and loved ones (Nyatanga, 2018). It would also be remiss at this point if we did not discuss the work of Dr Elizabeth Kübler-Ross (Kübler Ross and Kessler, 2014), who identified the five stages of grief: (1) denial; (2) anger; (3) bargaining; (4) depression; (5) acceptance (Figure 6.2). Kübler-Ross said these stages are useful in describing and framing loss, but it must also be noted that not all individuals go through all of these stages and not necessarily in any prescribed order. In her book *On Death and Dying*, she wrote: 'The dying patient's problems come to an end, but the family's problems go on' (Kübler-Ross, 1970: 160). Reading the work of Kübler-Ross is recommended to all those who care for palliative and end of life patients.

Bereavement

Although bereavement can be said to be an individual experience and that we may all experience it in different ways, research has shown that there tend to be three contextualised experiences of people who are dealing with the death of a loved one: (1) the huge gap and void in our lives after the death of a loved one; (2) extreme acute grief; (3) the uncertain trajectory of grieving to the recovery period (Wilson et al., 2016). The other important aspect of grief for most individuals is regret, the regret of having not done things differently while their loved one was alive; this is usually centred around the lack of time spent with the dying or dead loved one (Coelho and Barbosa, 2017). If there are any problems, dysfunctions or concerns within family dynamics these are usually magnified within family groups if a loved one is dying or has died. Grief, loss and bereavement does not just happen after the death of a loved one but is also part of accepting the palliative diagnosis, the deterioration and care for someone we love. There is a grief and loss response in the anticipation of death, as an individual realises and understands that a loved one has an advanced and irreversible disease (Coelho and Barbosa, 2017). The level that individuals experience grief during the dying phase of their loved one has a direct link to communication, in particular how clinicians communicate information about physical deterioration and symptom treatment (Nielsen et al., 2017). This information again highlights, the importance of the good communication skills between paramedics and the patient's loved ones in the dying phase to reduce the burden of grief for family members in the future.

How comfortable are you coping and communicating with patients, carers and their loved ones in the dying phase? Look at an adapted version of Bugen's 'coping

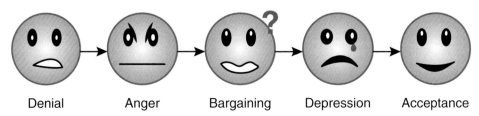

| Denial | Anger | Bargaining | Depression | Acceptance |

Figure 6.2 Five stages of grief

with death' scale below and decide how many of the statements you would answer yes to.

- I am aware of the emotions that are characteristics of grief.
- I can put words to my gut-level feelings about death and dying.
- I will be able to cope with my own future losses.
- I know how to listen to others, including dying patients.
- I can help someone with their thoughts and feelings about death and dying.
- I would be able to talk to a friend or family member about their death.
- I can lessen the anxiety of those around me when the topic of death and dying is discussed.

(Bugen, 1979)

Grief and Loss

The symptoms of grief are vast and multifaceted in their presentation, and they include not only psychological aspects but physical, emotional and spiritual manifestations:

- Physical symptoms:
  - loss of appetite
  - sleep disturbances
  - lethargy
  - exacerbation of illness
  - chest pain
  - a feeling of being hollow/emptiness.
- Emotional symptoms:
  - despair
  - guilt
  - anger
  - depression
  - loneliness.
- Cognitive symptoms:
  - preoccupation with thoughts of the deceased
  - feeling a physical presence of the deceased

- ■ finding it hard to concentrate

- ■ hopelessness.

- ● Behavioural symptoms:

  - ■ crying

  - ■ irritation

  - ■ anger

  - ■ tiredness

  - ■ increased intake of alcohol, medication or drugs.

- ● Social symptoms:

  - ■ social withdrawal

  - ■ changes in existing relationships

  - ■ revaluation of current social status and relationships.

- ● Spiritual symptoms:

  - ■ reflection on personal religious and spiritual perspectives

  - ■ a need for meaning/reflection and reasoning of events.

(Adapted from Machin, 2009)

Do Our Own Beliefs and Views About Death Affect Our Clinical Practice?

A German study looked at the influences of personal religious beliefs on clinical end of life decisions of a total of 429 paramedics, of whom 25.3% described themselves as non-believers, 10.1% as having strong religious beliefs, and 64.6% as moderately believing. The research concluded that paramedics who described themselves as more religious were more likely to transport a patient with an advance directive to hospital than leave them at home and also to think that death is not a natural part of life (Leibold et al., 2018). However, the study also concluded that the strongest correlation or influence on whether a paramedic would initiate hospitalisation of a patient at end of life or not was the paramedic's perception around their own competence in end of life care. This was connected to whether the paramedic had received end of life training or not, and the research stated that paramedics that received such education were better equipped to practice psychosocial care as well as clinical care for end of life patients and their families (Leibold et al., 2018). In summary, a paramedic's own personal religious beliefs can affect how they make clinical decisions for end of life patients, but other factors such as clinical experience and education are far more influential. The results of this research are congruent with other studies exploring the attitudes of paramedics to treating patients holistically at end of life (Kirk et al., 2017; O'Meara et al., 2017; Stone et al., 2009).

Key Points

- Is there a DNACPR order?

- Is there an advance care plan?

- Where is the patient's preferred place of care?

- Has anticipatory medication been prescribed? Is the anticipatory medication effective? If not, do you need to contact the on-call GP to review rather than take the patient to hospital?

- Is this patient known to the hospice? If this patient is not known, you, the paramedic, can refer to the community palliative care team.

- You, the paramedic, can ring the local hospice for advice on symptom control or any other issues, regardless of whether the end of life patient is known to them or not. This service is available 24 hours a day.

- Remember the factors that influence a 'good death' at home.

- Communication – have you explained to the patient and the family about symptom control and the rationale behind symptoms manifestation, e.g. noisy breathing?

- Listening – listen to the fears and concerns of the patient and their family.

- If the patient dies, spend time with the family to make sure they know who to call and inform.

- Remember, how you, the paramedic, behave after the death of the patient seriously affects the grieving process of the family. If you show compassion and give time, the family are more likely to perceive the death in positive terms, whereas if you are rushed and non-communicative towards the family, you may predispose them to complicated grief as opposed to a normal grief response.

- It's OK for you as a paramedic to feel upset and emotional about looking after patients at end of life. Look after yourself – you are a paramedic, but you are also a human being that is in a profession where you must look after patients experiencing the worst time in their lives, and that will affect you emotionally.

- Seek help from counselling, occupational health, friends, family and colleagues if you feel you need support. Seeking help is acting professionally and not a sign of weakness; seeking help will increase your professional resilience as a paramedic and enables you to do your job well.

- Remember that you, as a paramedic, can make a positive and invaluable difference in end of life care.

Case Studies

 Case Study 1

Mohamed is a 64-year-old man who was diagnosed with a glioblastoma two years ago. After undergoing surgery, radiation and chemotherapy he was in remission until his tumour reoccurred two months ago. During his latest admission it was decided that his brain tumour reoccurrence is inoperable, and he knows he has a palliative care status. During his stay in hospital Mohamed deteriorated and the decision was made with him and his family to discharge him home, so he could die at home in his preferred place of care. Mohamed has been discharged home with anticipatory medication, a DNAR, and a referral to the community palliative care team who will visit the day after discharge. Mohamed has a care package in place; carers visit three times a day to help with personal hygiene and feeding, although the family do a lot of care themselves.

Mohamed lives with his wife Saanvi who is 65 years old and is in good health. She is a retired social worker. They have two daughters: Aisha, who is 30 years old and who has her own family and has moved out, and Charita, who is 24 years old and still lives at home. Both daughters have been staying with their father, particularly overnight, to support their mother Saanvi.

Mohamed was discharged late last night and over the past eight hours he has become progressively lethargic and confused and appears to be actively dying. It is now 04.00.

Mohamed's breathing has slowed and he is gurgling; he is difficult to rouse. His wife, daughters and extended family (two brothers and their wives) have gathered around his bedside, in the front room of Mohamed's house. Although his wife and daughters are fully aware that Mohamed has been discharged home to die, they are very upset about his noisy breathing and think 'Mohamed is choking to death', so they have called 999 for help.

- How are you going to reassure Mohamed and his family?
- What do you think clinically is happening to Mohamed?
- What part of the dying process is this?
- Are there anticipatory medications that might help with this situation?
- DNAR?
- Have the palliative care team visited; if not, when are they visiting?
- Are you able to treat Mohamed and leave him in his preferred place of care?

Case Study 2

Mrs Stuart is an 85-year-old woman with pancreatic cancer. She is a known palliative care patient; she and her family are aware of her poor prognosis. She has decided that her preferred place of death is home and she has a DNAR order.

Mrs Stuart is at home. The community palliative care team and her GP are aware that she is at the end stage of her disease and she is actively dying. She has been visited by the district nurse today to recharge her syringe driver and has also been visited by her community palliative clinical nurse specialist from the hospice. Mrs Stuart rapidly deteriorates throughout the day. At 21.00 the family call 999 and request an ambulance as they become more and more distressed by Mrs Stuart's deteriorating condition.

You, the paramedic team, arrive at the house at 21.15. In the house are Mrs Stuart's elderly husband Fred, who is 87 years old and frail in appearance, and Mrs Stuart's two daughters – Maureen, 53 years old and Claire, 47 years old – as well as two grown up grandchildren, Harry, who is 27 years old and his sister Jessica, who is 23 years old.

You are met at the door by Harry, who shows you to the front room, which has been set up for Mrs Stuart to be looked after in. Mrs Stuart is in a hospital bed with her husband sitting at her side holding her hand. The rest of the family are cramped into the same room, including Sally the spaniel.

It is obvious to you that Mrs Stuart has just died, but you are not sure if the family realise this.

- What are you going to say to family members?
- Do you need to separate family members, into different rooms?
- Do you need to do any observations or vital signs?
- What authorities do you notify?
- What are the legal, moral and professional responsibilities in this scenario?

Case Study 3

Carol is a 45-year-old woman with lung, bone and liver metastasis. Carol is married to Tim and they live at home with their two teenage sons, Aron, 15 years old, and Dan, 13 years old. Carol has recently been in hospital with exacerbation of her shortness of breath. During her admission she was diagnosed with disease progression and her prognosis has been described to her and her husband and sons as she has 'short weeks'. Based on her poor prognosis, Carol has decided to be discharged home to spend her last weeks with her husband and sons. She has a DNAR, she has anticipatory medication in the house and is known to the community palliative care team at the hospice. She has been reviewed by them at 10.00 this morning as she has increased pain. Carol now has been commenced on a syringe driver with 30 mg of morphine over 24 hours, and 40 mg of metoclopramide over 24 hours in situ.

It is now 20.00 and Carol is agitated, distressed and confused; her breathing pattern has changed and is a combination of slow and rapid breathing. Her husband Tim has become very anxious and has dialled 999 requesting emergency help. Carol is seeking constant reassurance from her husband when you attend that she is not going to have to go to hospital. Her two sons are in the room as well, trying to comfort their mum.

- What are you going to say to Carol?
- What are going you to say to Tim?
- What are you going to say to Aron and Dan?
- What do you think is happening?
- Do you need to do any observations or vital signs?
- Is there any anticipatory medication that's appropriate to use?
- Do you need advice from any specialist team?
- Can you treat Carol at home, so she achieves her preferred place of care?

✳ Case Study 4

Adam is a 28-year-old man with metastatic melanoma, with metastases in his liver, bone and brain. He first had melanoma five years ago and at that time thought he was curative. He recently collapsed while playing tennis after injuring his arm. At the hospital he was scanned and diagnosed with a pathological fracture of humerus and, in addition, metastases were found in his liver and brain. Adam is single and lives with his mother, an occupational therapist at the local hospital; Adam's father died when Adam was 5 years old.

Adam has decided that he wants to be cared for at home, where he lives with his mum Brenda. He really hates hospital because of his previous cancer treatment when he was 23 years old. He also knows a lot of medics at the hospital socially because of his mother's job. Adam's prognosis has been explained to him as four to six weeks at best, but could be shorter as he has multiple brain metastases. He has received counselling while in hospital, he has a DNAR and is under the care of the palliative care team. Adam has anticipatory medication at home, which are injectables, but he hasn't used them as he is currently able to take oral medication. Adam and his mum have refused a care package. Adam's mum Brenda has taken time off work to care for Adam. Brenda did this for her husband and will do the same for her son.

Adam was visited by the clinical nurse specialist at midday yesterday and he reported that his symptoms were maintained on his oral medication. It is now 03.00 and Adam has been vomiting for the past two hours; as result of this he has been unable to take his oral medication. He is very distressed and in pain. His mother Brenda has called 999 asking for help.

- How are you going to reassure Adam?
- How are you going to reassure Brenda?
- How are you going to treat Adam's vomiting?
- How are you going to treat Adam's pain?
- How are you going to treat Adam's distress and agitation?
- Do you need specialist advice? Where from?
- Do you need to do vital signs?
- Are you able to treat Adam at home?

References

Albert RH (2017). End-of-life care: managing common symptoms. *American Family Physician*, 95(6): 356–361.

Armitage E and Jones C (2017). Paramedic attitudes towards DNACPR orders. *Journal of Paramedic Practice*, 9(10): 445–452.

Bayatrizi Z (2014). Death in a global age. *Canadian Journal of Sociology*, 39(2): 283–285.

Bone AE et al. (2018). What is the impact of population ageing on the future provision of end-of-life care? Population-based projections of place of death. *Palliative Medicine*, 32(2): 329–336.

Bugen L (1979). State anxiety effects on counselor perceptions of dying stages. *Journal of Counseling Psychology*, 26(1): 89–91.

Coelho A and Barbosa A (2017). Family anticipatory grief: an integrative literature review. *American Journal of Hospital Palliative Care*, 34: 774–785.

Collis E and Al-Qurainy R. (2013). Care of the dying patient in the community. *BMJ*, 347: f4085.

Department of Health (2013). *More Care, Less Pathway. A Review of the Liverpool Care Pathway*. London: DoH, 2013.

Dickman A (2012). *Drugs in Palliative Care*. Oxford: Oxford University Press.

Dickman A and Schneider J (2016). *The Syringe Driver: Continuous Subcutaneous Infusions in Palliative Care*. Oxford: Oxford University Press.

Ellershaw JE and Lakhani M (2013). Best care for the dying patient. *BMJ*, 347: f4428.

Finucane AM et al. (2017). The experiences of caregivers of patients with delirium, and their role in its management in palliative care settings: an integrative literature review. *Psycho-Oncology*, 26(3): 291.

Galiana L (2019). A brief measure for the assessment of competence in coping with death: the coping with death scale short version. *Journal of Pain and Symptom Management*, 57(2): 209–215.

Gannon C (2019). 70 Systematic review on the doctrine of double effect within palliative care. *BMJ Supportive and Palliative Care*, 9(Suppl 1): A34.

Hoare S et al. (2018). Ambulance staff and end-of-life hospital admissions: a qualitative interview study. *Palliative Medicine*, 32(9): 1465–1473.

Hodgkinson S et al. (2016). Care of dying adults in the last days of life. *Clinical Medicine (London, England)*, 16(3): 254–258.

Holdsworth LM (2015). Bereaved carers' accounts of the end of life and the role of care providers in a 'good death': a qualitative study. *Palliative Medicine*, 29(9): 834–841.

JRCALC and AACE (2019). *JRCALC Clinical Guidelines 2019*. Bridgwater: Class Professional Publishing.

Kastbom L, Milberg A and Karlsson M (2017). A good death from the perspective of palliative cancer patients. (Original Article). *Supportive Care in Cancer*, 25(3): 933.

Kirk A et al. (2017). Paramedics and their role in end-of-life care: perceptions and confidence. *Journal of Paramedic Practice*, 9(2): 71–79.

Kübler-Ross E (1970). *On Death and Dying*. New York, NY: Collier Books/Macmillan Publishing Co.

Kübler-Ross E and Kessler D (2014). *On Grief and Grieving: Finding the Meaning of Grief through the Five Stages of Loss*. London: Simon & Schuster.

Lawley H and Hewison A (2017). An integrative literature review exploring the clinical management of delirium in patients with advanced cancer. *Journal of Clinical Nursing*, 26: 4172–4183.

Leibold A et al. (2018). Is every life worth saving: does religion and religious beliefs influence paramedics' end-of-life decision-making? A prospective questionnaire-based investigation. *Indian Journal of Palliative Care*, 24(1): 9.

Lindqvist O et al. (2013). Four essential drugs needed for quality care of the dying: a Delphi-study based international expert consensus opinion. *Journal of Palliative Medicine*, 16(1): 38–43.

Machin L (2009). *Working with Loss and Grief: A New Model for Practitioners*. London: SAGE.

Meier EA et al. (2016). Defining a good death (successful dying): literature review and a call for research and public dialogue. *The American Journal of Geriatric Psychiatry: Official Journal of the American Association for Geriatric Psychiatry*, 24(4): 261–271.

National Institute for Health and Care Excellence (2020). *NICE guidance*. Available at: https://www.nice.org.uk/guidance.

Nielsen MK et al. (2017). Preloss grief in family caregivers during end-of-life cancer care: a nationwide population-based cohort study. *Psycho-Oncology*, 26(12): 2048–2056.

Nyatanga B. (2018). Loss, grief and bereavement: an inescapable link in palliative care. *British Journal of Community Nursing*, 23(2): 70.

Olausson J and Ferrell BR (2013). Care of the body after death: nurses' perspectives of the meaning of post-death patient care. (CNE Article) (Report). *Clinical Journal of Oncology Nursing*, 17(6): 647.

O'Meara P, Furness S and Gleeson R (2017). Educating paramedics for the future: a holistic approach. *Journal of Health and Human Services Administration*, 40(2): 219–251.

Parkinson M (2015). Pain: highlighting the law and ethics of pain relief in end-of-life patients. *Journal of Paramedic Practice*, 7(7): 344–349.

Pettifer A and Bronnert R (2013). End of life care in the community: the role of ambulance clinicians. *Journal of Paramedic Practice*, 5(7): 394-399.

Rayment C and Ward J (2011). Care of the dying patient in hospital. *British Journal of Hospital Medicine (London, England: 2005)*, 72(8): 451–455.

Read S and Macbride-Stewart S (2018). The 'good death' and reduced capacity: a literature review. *Mortality*, 23(4): 381–395.

Regnard C et al. (2011). So, farewell then, doctrine of double effect. *BMJ*, 343(7818): 274.

Reid VL et al. (2017). A systematically structured review of biomarkers of dying in cancer patients in the last months of life: an exploration of the biology of dying. *PLoS ONE*, 12(4): e0175123–e0175123.

Royal College of Physicians (2016). CEEU. *National Care of the Dying Audit for Hospitals*. London: RCP.

Ruijs CDM et al. (2013). Symptoms, unbearability and the nature of suffering in terminal cancer patients dying at home: a prospective primary care study. *BMC Family Practice*, 14: 201.

Steindal SA et al. (2011). Pain control at the end of life: A comparative study of hospitalized cancer and noncancer patients. *Scandinavian Journal of Caring Sciences*, 25(4): 771–779.

Stone SC et al. (2009). Paramedic knowledge, attitudes, and training in end-of-life care. *Prehospital and Disaster Medicine*, 24(6): 529.

Thompson J (2018). Opioids and cancer pain. *International Journal of Palliative Nursing*, 24(11): 536–538.

van der Werff GFM, Paans W and Nieweg RMB (2012). Hospital nurses' views of the signs and symptoms that herald the onset of the dying phase in oncology patients. *International Journal of Palliative Nursing*, 18(3): 143–149.

Waldrop DP, McGinley JM and Clemency B (2018). The nexus between the documentation of end-of-life wishes and awareness of dying: a model for research, education and care. *Journal of Pain and Symptom Management*, 55(2): 522–529.

Wallerstedt B et al. (2012). Identification and documentation of persons being in palliative phase regardless of age, diagnosis and places of care, and their use of a sitting service at the end of life. *Scandinavian Journal of Caring Sciences*, 26(3): 561–568.

Wilson DM, Macleod R and Houttekier D (2016). Examining linkages between bereavement grief intensity and perceived death quality: qualitative findings. *OMEGA – Journal of Death and Dying*, 74(2): 260–274.

Yun Y et al. (2018). Priorities of a 'good death' according to cancer patients, their family caregivers, physicians, and the general population: a nationwide survey. *Supportive Care in Cancer*, 26(10): 3479–3488.

Chapter 7

Ethics

Marlon Stiell

Introduction

Ethics form an important and essential part of care in all settings. Ambulance trusts and ambulance clinicians increasingly recognise the importance of ethical decision making in the role of maintaining patient autonomy to improve healthcare outcomes (Waldrop, 2014; Brady, 2013; Wiese et al., 2012). There has been a rise in the number of people seeking assistance from emergency services for a range of increasingly complex and chronic life-limiting conditions, including those who are older and experience end of life and palliative care interventions (Evans et al., 2017; Sampson et al., 2018; Voss et al., 2017). To manage the changing demands in emergency and primary care, paramedics are being equipped with an increasing number of clinical interventions, including paramedic prescribing. The increase in clinical skills for ambulance staff is in line with reorganisation of emergency and primary care services (Maruthappu et al., 2014) to better manage patients in the community or aged care facilities (Leong and Crawford, 2018). Emergency situations do not always allow time for consideration of all the factors present, such as advance care planning, or to devise a plan which suits all (Tirkkonen et al., 2016).

A recent report commissioned by Public Health England (2015), *National End of Life Care Intelligence Network: Ambulance Data Project for End of Life Care*, investigated some of the problems ambulance staff may experience when clinically assessing if a person is in receipt of end of life or palliative care. While ambulance clinicians are confident with 'do not attempt cardiopulmonary resuscitation' (DNACPR), events that do not require immediate clinical intervention are more challenging and prone to ambiguity. In the same report Public Health England (2015) observed that 18% of patients who were admitted to hospital had accompanying documentation or had been clearly identified as being terminally ill or near the end of their life. Eight per cent of the medical records reviewed found the information to be unclear in that the person may be terminally ill or approaching the end of their life. The majority of the medical records sampled (63%, 270 patients) did not include information which identified the person as being terminally ill or approaching the end of life. This potentially presents a problem for staff who come into contact with persons without the information needed to help decide on the most appropriate course of action, and presents a potential cause of conflict with family, carers and healthcare professionals when determining the best course of action.

It is, therefore, extremely important that ambulance clinicians possess a good understanding of ethics and their applications in practice before encountering complex clinical and social situations where patients have been identified as nearing the end of their life or in receipt of palliative care (Brady, 2014). The intention of this chapter is to present some of the key issues regarding ethics in our treatment of those requiring interventions at end of life care or in receipt of palliative care. Medical ethics, or bioethics, can be seen as the practical application of moral philosophy to the clinical practice environment. This can be defined as 'the analytical activity in which the concepts, assumptions, beliefs, attitudes, emotions, reasons and arguments underlying medico-moral decision making are examined critically' (Macnair, 1999). So, ethics when applied in healthcare set out to provide a framework to help resolve matters of health when faced with competing choices or difficult decisions (Avery, 2017). There are a number of debates and key issues within ethics relevant to a discussion of end of life/palliative care patients; for example, the belief that it is wrong to allow a person in pain to continue to suffer, and questions around how we should treat persons with cognitive impairments and how can we gain consent when a person is incapacitated and wishes to end their life. Another way of seeing these issues would be to consider the ways in which we apply the primary survey to a range of patient presentations with little variation; likewise, we should aim to achieve a type of consistency with our ethical decision making. In making ethical decisions we must consider the types of interactions we have with patients. Our aim should be to foster a positive relationship with the patient's carers/families and other healthcare professionals to achieve ethical and clinical interventions that enhance and prolong life (Mason et al., 2016). We cannot discuss all ethical issues; therefore, the focus of this chapter will be on the ethical principles incorporated into the HCPC *Standards of Conduct Performance and Ethics* (HCPC, 2016), *Standards of Proficiency* (HCPC, 2014) and the *Mental Capacity Act 2005* (Department of Health, 2005). These standards and acts of legislation provide a framework for ethical decision making in clinical practice.

Summary of the Mental Capacity Act 2005

The *Mental Capacity Act (MCA) 2005*, enacted in 2007 (DoH, 2005), is legislation which requires all healthcare professionals to consider patient autonomy, informed consent, capacity to consent, decisions made by surrogate or best interest decisions and careful handling of sensitive information. The act applies to all healthcare interactions where the patient is over the age of 16 and experiences a loss in capacity to make decisions regarding their own health. Persons over the age of 18 who wish to formalise their wishes in the event of being incapacitated may also do so with the support of healthcare professionals and significant others.

The MCA's main purpose is to support individuals and their families when the recipient of care lacks capacity. There are five principles that underpin the application of the MCA in clinical practice. These are:

1. **A presumption of capacity** – the person in receipt of care is assumed to have capacity to consent to treatment.

2. **Individuals being supported to make their own decisions** – healthcare professionals should support patients to make decisions regarding their care, without duress or coercion.

3. **Unwise decisions** – it is a patient's right to make unwise decisions regarding their health if they have the capacity to do so.

4. **Best interests** – decisions made regarding the health of a person who lacks capacity must be done with reference to their best interests.

5. **Less restrictive options** – the healthcare professional involved should consider the effect of any intervention and try to ensure that decisions or actions cause least harm or impact on an individual's rights and freedoms. It might be the case that no action is the best course.

Within the MCA there are two tests to ascertain the capacity of a person:

- 1st Stage: Does the person have an impairment or disturbance of the mind or brain? If 'yes', then proceed to the 2nd Stage of the test. If 'no', then it must be concluded that the person has capacity.

- 2nd Stage: Does the impairment or disturbance mean that the person is unable to make the decision in question at the time it needs to be made?

(DoH, 2005)

To ensure that ambulance staff comply with the MCA, they should assemble the relevant information, which should be in a format that the patient can understand and retain long enough to make the decision, for example using non-technical language, and where possible have a family member or carer present to provide support.

The patient must have a means of communicating their wishes regarding the decisions they have made. If they are unable to meet these requirements, then they are deemed not to have capacity.

✴ Case Study 1

A paramedic crew are called to attend a 78-year-old man, who is unwell having refused fluids for the past two days. On arrival at the patient's home a family member is present.

The patient appears limp and semi-conscious..He is unable to answer questions clearly and appears confused at times. He does not maintain eye contact with the attending paramedic. He is offered a drink but refuses to suck on a straw. Further attempts to provide the patient with water are met with refusal. The last attempt is pushed away by the patient. You notice the patient wince in pain. You are informed that the patient has a necrotic pressure sore on his back. There is no documentary evidence of any care plan in the home.

- Does this patient have capacity? (In answering this question consider the likely response to 1st and 2nd Stage questions for a person who is semi-conscious).
- What are the treatment decisions at this point? (Can you gain consent from a patient who cannot retain information, is semi-conscious but is able to refuse fluids?)
- On what basis will these decisions be made?
- Can you suggest a more suitable solution than the emergency department? Or is the emergency department the only alternative?

Ethical Theories

Deontology and Utility

Two ethical approaches that form part of the basis for ethical decisions taken in healthcare are the ideas of Emmanuel Kant (Deontology) and Jeremy Bentham's and John Mills' Utility (otherwise known as Consequentialism).

Kant's ideas are based on several principles. Firstly, these ideas are derived from the tradition of western philosophy, which is very different from eastern ideas regarding human rights and moral actions. Kant assumed that humans will act or behave in a rational manner. Rational thoughts are as a result of the human free will and an intention to maximise good outcomes (Upton, 2011).

Kant argues that a set of universal principles may govern situations where the outcome is unsure or ambiguous. The action itself and the rightness of this action should be foremost in our thoughts when deciding what to do. Kant stated that we should act only in accordance with that maxim, through which you can at the same time will, that it become a universal law. Kant is arguing that good outcomes are morally right outcomes; therefore, the actions which lead to good outcomes should become universal law and be applied in all circumstances. For example, we should not murder our neighbour. Often called duty-based ethics, we act not because of the consequences to ourselves or the other party involved, but because it is the right thing to do (Kant, 1996).

Consider the following. We may take someone who is unwell to hospital to receive medical care when they lack capacity. They may wish to remain at home to receive care, which you cannot provide. Our processes for working as ambulance staff are to preserve and promote life, so to leave someone at home who is unwell goes against a developed system and way of working. In such a scenario the course of action is clear in that this person should be conveyed to hospital, as it is the right thing to do even if the outcome is emotional distress and anxiety for the patient and family (Upton, 2011).

Duty-based ethics are important in healthcare and human rights, as they emphasise the value of every human being. Each person should be treated with equal respect and dignity. This idea of equality and dignity has become a cornerstone in the way we view human rights. The duty to do the right thing against your self-interest is important, in particular when the needs of the individual appear to be in conflict with those who hold the majority view.

Often presented in contrast to deontology is utility or consequentialism. This is the idea that we should behave with reference to the consequences of our actions. An action or behaviour is morally correct if it results in the generation of a positive outcome, i.e. maximises the good obtained from a circumstance and if this good outweighs the potential negative outcomes. In other words, we should always seek the best outcomes for ourselves and wider society. This view directs the individual to avoid pain and seek pleasure. There are several different formulations of utilitarianism; however, if you consider the previous example from a utilitarian view, you may decide not to take a person to hospital even when capacity is in doubt, as this may appease the carers and family members. Utilitarianism argues that our actions should lead to the greater good or the greatest good. Whichever action leads to the greatest happiness for all is the right action – in contrast to deontology we are considering the consequences of our actions when deciding (Roache, 2014).

Adopting either approach in isolation is problematic when weighing up the considerations involved in caring for complex patients and those in receipt of palliative or end of life care.

Critique of Deontology and Utility

It will not always follow that taking someone to hospital is the right decision or that telling untruths is always wrong. Consider the following example of a conflict which may arise if we follow only deontological principles. One ethical circumstance that we should consider alongside capacity and autonomy of the individual is that of lying and persons with cognitive impairment.

Consider a circumstance where you are caring for a person with complex healthcare needs at the end stages of a debilitating and terminal illness who is cognitively impaired.

Imagine that the individual did not remember that a loved one had died some time ago, and that each time you break the news to them, they relive the news of the death as though it was for the first time, which it is for them, as their impairment gives them no memory of the event taking place. Here is an example of conflict between duty to be honest and to have integrity versus non-maleficence and to not cause harm (Tuckett, 2012).

In such circumstances where honesty and integrity are in conflict as in our example, deontologists are unable to propose a compromise, as actions are either right or wrong. Such an approach to ethical decision making is inflexible, particularly when caring for those in receipt of end of life interventions and treatments.

Utilitarian ideas may lead to harm being caused to individuals; for example, stealing is morally right if it increases the overall good for society. A utilitarian may argue that if the harm caused by lying results in a greater good, then lying is permissible. Again, this is an unsatisfactory solution not only because it goes against the need to be honest, but because it leads to inconsistent behaviour, as there will be circumstances where lying is clearly inappropriate.

Another difficulty with a strictly utilitarian approach is that we cannot be sure that a decision will lead to the greatest good or happiness – we can only see so far into the future and at some point it is difficult to determine cause and effect. One of the central concepts within both these theories is what constitutes happiness; however, understanding what happiness is in the circumstance where a person is nearing the end of their life can be difficult to determine.

Ethical Decision Making

One way of attempting to resolve the issues presented by deontological and utilitarian philosophies is principlism, as proposed by Beauchamp and Childress (2013), which consists of four components and is the ethical approach most frequently applied to the clinical practice environment. In this ethical approach, the autonomy of the patient is seen as a key concept within healthcare interactions. Autonomy is defined as the patient's right to choose or refuse treatment or interventions in his/her own life. The caveat of course is the patient's ability to understand information and consent to treatment.

Ambulance clinicians should advocate and promote the autonomy of any person they care for within the context of principlism; beneficence is the idea that healthcare professionals must promote the wellbeing of the patient and weigh the benefits of an action against the potential risks to a person.

Non-maleficence is the duty not to cause harm; that is not to say that harm is never possible. In the ambulance context harm is often caused for greater potential benefits, for example, the insertion of an intravenous cannula to deliver drugs. However, we should consider other ways in which we could intervene to reduce or eliminate harms in our practice.

Justice in healthcare is consideration of the available information to arrive at measured conclusions and fair decisions, which seek to represent objectivity in our decision making. In the pre-hospital context, this would be ensuring that treatment is not withheld, and all possible options are discussed. Patients and carers value the expertise that ambulance clinicians possess. One practical formulation of principlism is the process of gaining informed consent, which involves interpretation and discussion of sometimes complex medical conditions in terms that a lay person can understand. These types of encounters require a skilled person who can discuss the different complexities of each case (Sutherland et al., 2012). There is an assumption that gaining informed consent will automatically preserve patient rights and autonomy, by providing them with the opportunity to weigh up the potential harms and benefits to a particular treatment (Corrigan, 2003).

This can be problematic when we do not fully understand research methods or are not in a position to interpret the results of a study to be fully able to discuss with our patients in terms they can readily understand at a time when they are vulnerable mentally and physically (Delany, 2007).

We should also consider that family members called upon to make complex care decisions may experience stress and post-traumatic stress disorder, e.g. guilt about the decisions made, and lingering doubt regarding whether the right decisions were made (Wendler and Rid, 2011), so it is important that, where possible, ethical thinking is explicit and involves all parties.

Often philosophical ideas are presented as opposites and incompatible. If you review the standards for performance and ethics (HCPC, 2016), many of Kant's and Bentham's ideas are contained within; for example, 'You must treat service users and carers as individuals, respecting their privacy and dignity' (deontological) and 'You must take all reasonable steps to reduce the risk of harm to service users' (utilitarian). In reality we use both deontological and utilitarian principles; we act depending upon the circumstances and our experience, but ethical principles are important in guiding our behaviour to achieve positive health outcomes for patients and their families.

Cross Cultural Values

There may be occasions where different cultural and religious values come into conflict. In all circumstances we must ensure that policy and practice conform to the law, which defines for ambulance clinicians the scope of treatment and potential liability in the end of life phase.

Culture and ethics can intersect along the same concepts contained within principlism, but the presentation in end of life care may vary. Using the example of truth-telling, we may encounter a circumstance where the patient is unaware that they are terminally unwell. The family or family member may have decided to conceal a diagnosis from the patient. The decision to disclose or withhold information is seen as a family process in some cultures. As a result of a shared decision-making process, which includes beneficence and non-maleficence, the emphasis is the group's decision to advocate in the best interests of the patient and family rather than give primacy to individual autonomy. This process has been described, conceptualised and understood as guided autonomy. The degree to which the concepts of principlism are adhered to depends upon the cultural context. Some cultures may rank beneficence above autonomy, hence the example that providing information of a terminal diagnosis may remove hope from a patient and cause harm. This type of thinking leads to the expectation that aggressive treatment should continue even when futile (Brown, 2014). Other studies have found that persons who have a strong religious belief often delay or deny the need to formulate any kind of advance planning in instances of a terminal diagnosis (van Wijmen et al., 2010).

Ambulance clinicians in these circumstances may find it challenging to consider and satisfy all parties to achieve a positive outcome (Murphy-Jones and Timmons, 2016).

Ohr et al. (2017) observed that people with Asian backgrounds were more likely to accept dying as a normal part of life, whereas 64% of Eastern Europeans and 53% of people from the Asia/Pacific region surveyed in their study believed that all efforts should be taken to avoid death, even in the context of a terminal diagnosis.

Cultural expectations and practices in Indian and Pakistani families often focus on the role of women. The expectation may be that women should take the role of primary caregiver, while the immediate family bear the financial cost. Other stresses will include psychosocial and physical burdens as a result of the care, and these are expected to be shared by both the immediate and extended family. There is a cultural expectation that patients will be, and prefer to be, treated at home rather than in hospital. This is also reflected in the care of older people with chronic conditions who require complex care (Lambert, et al., 2017; Ferri and Jacob, 2017). Indian families may also participate in a number of religious ceremonies and rituals as part of care, for example, drinking holy water and wearing jewellery believed to be fortuitous (Ramasamy Venkatasalu, 2018).

Religious practices including those of Christian, Islamic and Jewish faiths contain many of the ideas and concepts that relate to principlism. The right to life is seen as unconditional in Islam, so interventions that may harm (non-maleficence) or limit life would not be considered. Conversely treatments that prolong life are seen as beneficial, as every additional day of life is of value (Westra et al., 2009). Therefore, in keeping with Catholicism and Judaism, interventions and treatments that prolong suffering and pain at the end of life or in palliative care should be avoided. The role of suffering has both positive and negative connotations in end of life care situations. The role of duty in Islam provides obligations for family members and ensures family members and loved ones are supported and cared for; for example, it is expected that children will care for their parents (Choong, 2015).

✚ Case Study 2

A paramedic crew attend an 84-year-old woman with leukaemia. English is her second language (she is from Malaysia). You have been called due to the patient experiencing pain in her chest, back and knees. The patient discloses that she has a strong belief in god, which has been strengthened despite her recent terminal diagnosis. The patient is at home with her daughter. Her daughter says she has been trying to get her mother to eat and rest, but she is not sure if her mother has been taking her prescribed medications. The patient sees these medications as 'strong medicine', so although they would help alleviate her symptoms, taking these strong medications may also hasten the end of life or signal that she is near the end of life.

You describe to the patient via the daughter what these medications are for, including side effects and the benefits of taking these medications. The patient refuses to take medications with side effects as they would affect her relationship with her daughter, and it will not help her get better.

- How can you manage this situation?
- Does this patient have capacity?
- Can we consider the role of beliefs and culture to ensure we choose the least restrictive option?

Discussion of Case Study 2

Within Catholicism, human life is also seen as a gift from God and to be preserved. However, this does not mean that life should be maintained at all costs when it is clear that an individual is suffering. Pain should be alleviated when possible, in particular in end of life care, even when there is the possibility that analgesia may ultimately shorten the person's life (known as double effect). Religious interpretations of truth-telling in Catholicism and end of life scenarios state that a patient should be informed of their condition unless they have expressed a desire not to know. With regards to initiating or withdrawal of treatment, the interpretation is in the intention to cause harm. If withdrawing treatment leads to alleviating suffering and pain, then this is acceptable; however, if the intention is to hasten death, then this is viewed as contrary to Catholic teaching (Clarfield et al., 2003).

Jewish religious practices also place emphasis on guided autonomy. However, the emphasis in Jewish medical ethics is on 'duties, obligations, commandments, and reciprocal responsibility' (Steinberg, 2003). Patients are duty bound to see doctors regarding their health problems to prevent ill health and deterioration, while doctors are duty bound to provide help in all circumstances (Steinberg, 2003)

Treatment that is undertaken is made with reference to religious scripture, often interpreted by a rabbi, but that is not to say that an individual cannot decide on their own treatment (Greenberger, 2015). The decisions taken are not only made with reference to the health of the person but the effect on their family. The view may be taken that advance planning of treatments and intervention to prepare for the end of life is something that only God is able to decide: 'Causing life to end either directly by an act of commission or indirectly by an act of omission is not properly within a human being's authority' (Greenberger, 2015). Another way to frame this would be that autonomy is understood in the secular sense; however, devout Jews will limit their own decisions and choices to comply with religious scripture (Kinzbrunner, 2004). This will have implications for formulation of advance directives as they may not be considered or include detail of interventions which might be seen to hasten death. Yet this does not mean that patients should continue to suffer in order to prolong life (Glick, 2016) when in fact Jewish scholars agree that we should do all we can to alleviate suffering and pain in these circumstances (Jotkowitz and Zivotofsky, 2010).

The aim of summarising some of the different cultural and religious beliefs that exist is to demonstrate that these provide a basis for discussion regarding the needs and desires of patients and families who are caring for people at the end of life. Despite different cultural practices, there are a number of ethical principles which form common ground for beginning any discussion, including autonomy of the patient and/or family to make decisions, not to cause harm (alleviation of pain and suffering), compassion, to promote wellbeing where possible, fairness, equal access to resources, and avoiding inequalities (Bossaert et al., 2015; The Human Rights Act, 1998; Zieske and Abbott, 2011). These situations are not always easily resolved; however, along with emphasis on communication, one way forward is through advance directives and advance care planning.

Advance Directives and Advance Care Planning

To begin, it is important to distinguish advance directives from advance care planning. Advance directives (AD) are documents that formally convey an individual's wishes about medical decisions to be made in the event that he or she loses decision-making capacity. In contrast, advance care planning refers to a process that involves preparing for future medical treatments and interventions that may be required in the event of the individual being unconscious or lacking capacity, and provides direction for medical practitioners, family and carers in what actions are required (van Wijmen et al., 2010).

Advance care plans (ACPs) are documents typically used where a person is assessed as being in the last months of life (12 months or fewer). ACPs can be defined as follows:

> Advance care planning is a voluntary process of discussion and review to help an individual who has capacity to anticipate how their condition may affect them in the future and, if they wish, set on record: choices about their care and treatment and/or an advance decision to refuse a treatment in specific circumstances, so that these can be referred to by those responsible for their care or treatment (whether professional staff or family carers) in the event that they lose capacity to decide once their illness progresses.

> (National End of Life Care Programme, 2017)

Advance directives reflect and consider the choices made by a patient and they convey what to expect from end of life and palliative care, which treatments they do not wish to endure and which they are willing to have administered. This is also providing the person making the advance directive a degree of control over their medical care and their future, obtaining guarantees that they will die in the way they have chosen (Yen et al., 2018)

Planning may also include and consider other values, for example, cultural and religious beliefs as previously summarised. In our interventions we can use these plans to mitigate any conflict that may arise when discussing the needs of the patient, while assuring the patient that you will try to facilitate their wishes. Details of the potential impact of treatment and non-treatment will be included, for example, the effect these interventions may have on quality of life. Finally, in the event of the person experiencing a loss of capacity, the advance directive will provide information on a nominated advocate (Levi and Green, 2010).

Directives, also known as living wills, identify situations in which the patient would or would not want specified treatments. For example, a patient's directive might state that 'if I am permanently unconscious or terminally ill, I would not want to undergo cardiopulmonary resuscitation' (Bossaert et al., 2015).

Documents vary in terms of the scenarios described and the specificity of the different treatments. Some documents use general terms, such as 'aggressive care'; however, living wills may also contain information of circumstances where an unwell person wishes to have clinical interventions and treatment.

In contrast, advance care planning (ACP) provides specificity as a person's illness progresses and it becomes clearer which possible circumstances they might face at the end of their life. ACPs are a useful starting point where there is difficulty interpreting the wishes of a person, and can be used to make best-interest decisions.

ACPs may include DNACPR orders, and should be considered where resuscitation attempts will not be successful.

Although the circumstances in which DNACPR are used are expected to be clearly stated within an ACP, there are situations where ambulance staff feel they need to perform CPR. Rajagopal et al. (2016) observed that 1 in 10 patient resuscitations were influenced by whether bystander CPR was commenced within 15 minutes or not. The fact that CPR is being performed before arrival will result in the ambulance crew continuing resuscitation attempts unless it is clear efforts would be futile or there is evidence of a DNACPR order. Several studies have highlighted that ambulance staff clearly understand DNACPR orders; however, circumstances are complicated by the presence of family members and carers performing CPR when the ambulance crew arrives, with some staff feeling under pressure to continue CPR (Rajagopal et al., 2016; Moffat et al., 2019).

Some ambulance staff expressed challenges in interpreting DNACPR; for most, though, they were useful in determining the patient's wishes, deciding if a person should be transported to hospital and which interventions would be in keeping with the patient's wishes.

Armitage and Jones (2017) identified concerns that patients' general practitioners needed to be more involved in their care, in particular the discussions concerning treatment plans. There is evidence to suggest that part of the problem in interpreting the use of DNACPR is the lack of available resources outside office hours to inform decisions around care (Smythe et al., 2017). What is clear is that there has been insufficient and inconsistent education regarding the issue of end of life care for the families of patients and ambulance staff (Kirk et al., 2017)

In legal terms the *Mental Capacity Act* (DoH, 2005) requires ambulance staff to refer to ACPs in circumstances where informed consent is difficult to obtain. Some of the principles regarding end of life care contained within the act include the following:

- A person must have the capacity to take part in advance care planning at the time of documenting their wishes, concerns and desires, as well as discuss treatment options and make decisions. A person with a life-limiting illness should make these decisions without pressure or duress.

- Ambulance staff should be able to communicate effectively, with empathy and compassion.

- A person may not have an ACP as it is a voluntary process; therefore, if one is not present, the ambulance clinician must gain informed consent before starting any care.

- Ambulance staff must ensure adequate information is provided to patients and their families so that they may make informed decisions regarding their care.

- In circumstances where a person lacks capacity to make informed choices, best interest decisions can be made, and care planning must focus on determining their best interests and making decisions to protect these.

- Where an individual chooses to refuse care or treatment in the event of a loss of capacity, this refusal of care comes into effect where there is a clear loss of capacity.

- Patients and families are encouraged to regularly review the contents of any documents to ensure that they accurately reflect their desires and wishes.

- Help the family/carers to understand your role in this situation as well as their own.

These documents should be available to all those involved in the care of someone in receipt of end of life/palliative care, including those working in out-of-hours and emergency settings (National End of Life Care Programme, 2017).

✳ Case Study 3

A paramedic crew arrive at the home of a woman aged 66 with severe dementia. She is unable to communicate with you or carers on scene. The carer informs you that she cried out in pain while being transferred to a bed from a wheelchair. She appears to have a fractured femur in the right leg.

The patient appears to be in pain and grimaces and grinds her teeth. Her husband is at work. He gives permission over the phone for you to take his wife to hospital and to administer analgesia. You are unsure as he is not at home and when you previously tried to administer pain relief, she pulled her arm away. There is an advance directive in place, which states that in the event of a stroke or unconsciousness then no treatment should be given. The AD does not specify anything regarding the current circumstances.

- How will you manage this situation?

Discussion of Case Study 3

Advance directives are a useful tool in negotiating ethical problems encountered in practice, though they are not always able to resolve problems of an ethical nature. ADs need to be specific in scope and use of language as they could be open to unintended interpretations and consequences; for example, even if a document is specific, it will not be able to cover every possible outcome available for the individual (Detering et al., 2010).

In the case study the AD gives detail of some circumstances; however, there could be discord, as it does not specify dementia or a fracture. Disagreement on the best course of action can occur even when there is an acceptance of the current situation or diagnosis. Family members may re-interpret the content of the advance directive, and believe that the patient changed his or her mind, or that they would not refuse life-saving treatment and interventions (Alonso et al., 2017).

When a patient who has an advance directive lacks decision-making capacity and is seriously ill, the ambulance staff should discuss the situation with the named surrogate and other appropriate loved ones. Reviewing the advance directive, those involved should decide what they think the patient would have wanted under the current circumstances. People who are not used to working with advance directives often misunderstand these documents (Levi and Green, 2010). For example, an advance directive may state that life-sustaining treatment should be forgone, but mention only the scenario of permanent unconsciousness (Qureshi et al., 2013). If the patient under your care has experienced life-limiting illness but is not in a state of permanent unconsciousness, the document itself may not provide the required detail needed to proceed with the patient's wishes and treatment (Satyanarayana Rao, 2008).

Family members and ambulance clinicians may disagree on the concept of futility, when treatment is no longer effective and there is not a good chance of recovery. Some patients and their families may take the view that, in discussing the issue of advance directives, the discussion provides a type of consent to withdraw treatment, in particular in the presence of a terminal diagnosis.

Due to the often complex presentation of diseases, some ambulance staff find it difficult to identify if a person is dying, and if the current presentation is an expected part of the disease process (Waldrop, 2015). The lack of specificity in ADs means that, it is difficult to determine if a person requires intervention if they are choking, but also in the last stages of their ill health (Kirk, 2018).

There have been instances where advance directives have not accompanied patients to hospital or nursing homes. This may create additional problems when patients are not under the care of their regular doctor when they are hospitalised, and the hospital staff may not know about the existence of an advance directive (Pecanac et al., 2014).

In situations where there is a disagreement, it is helpful if advocates and ambulance clinicians can agree on the wishes of the patient and the reason why the advance directive was written in the first instance. Many medical conditions are treatable due to advances in medicine (Delany, 2008); however, loved ones or healthcare providers may disagree on the meaning of a 'reasonable chance of recovery', for example. In this case as well, it is helpful to try to focus decision makers on what they think the patient would have wanted (Iserson, 2006). Although it is best to gain a consensus of all the interested parties, especially about forgoing life-sustaining treatment, ultimately a named proxy has the final decision (Evans et al., 2012).

One such example is CPR. If it is clear that performing CPR will not work because the person is experiencing advanced symptoms and death is inevitable, there is an opportunity to explain to the family/carers that you may actually cause more harm (Caldwell, 2015)

Ambulance clinicians should be cautious in overriding the decisions made by advocates as advocates have been given authority by patients. People often write advance directives to relieve family members of the burden of decision making, as the patient may not have wanted a family member to undergo the distress involved in making on the spot decisions.

These conflicts within ADs are not easily resolved, and often result in transportation to acute care, in particular where diagnosis and symptoms do not suggest the end stages of life. However, this may be against the wishes of the patient and family.

Ethics in Practice: Best Interests, Autonomy, Consent and Capacity

When seeking to apply ethical principles to clinical practice, models have been developed to ensure consistency and objectivity in our interactions with our patients. The majority of our interactions are non-clinical in that they involve discussion, negotiation and joint decisions. A small number will involve interactions where our patients are unconscious or unable to consent, which will require us to act in their best interests (O'Neill, 2003).

Family members and carers call 999 in a panic as patients begin to suffer respiratory failure, with this being the most common reason for hospital admissions.

This suggests that these admissions could be avoided with better planning, and discussion of the expectation of medicine and care so that these patients could be better managed at home.

Where information about a person is incomplete or you are required to discuss the care of person with capacity, best interests process should be followed (as defined within the MCA 2005 Code of Practice, DoH 2005).

Best interest decisions are not easily defined. However, the process involves consultation with other healthcare professionals involved in the care of the patient, consideration of the relevant facts and circumstances, and consultation with the patient and their family/carers. It may involve a person who has lasting power of attorney (LPA). The scope of the LPA should be checked during consultation to ensure that its reach includes decisions regarding the health and social care of the patient. The person who has LPA should be appointed before the patient had lost capacity. Decisions made with reference to an individual holding the title of lasting power of attorney are considered acting in a person's best interests.

The aim of our interaction with patients and carers should be to arrive at a consensus that minimises deception or coercion, and where patients can decline treatment at any time without fear of repercussion (except of course possible negative health outcomes). Contemporary policy that helps to shape and direct end of life care faces a tension between end of life liability and the way in which palliative care is developing (Leadership Alliance for the Care of Dying People (LACDP), 2014).

✴ Case Study 4

A paramedic crew are called to a 44-year-old man with difficulty in breathing. On arrival you assess him and discover that he has terminal lung cancer. You offer him oxygen and a nebuliser, after which he immediately requests that you leave. He still appears breathless. There is an ACP in place, which states that in the event of respiratory arrest he is not to be resuscitated. His daughter is on scene and has lasting power of attorney.

- How will you manage this situation?
- Do you act in the best interest here or is this an example of an unwise decision?
- Who could you contact to assist with decisions regarding his care?

Discussion of Case Study 4

Ambulance education and training focuses on the acquisition of knowledge and skills to prevent deterioration of those who are acutely unwell or experience exacerbations of existing chronic conditions. The 'natural' disposition is to prevent deterioration in a patient, which partly explains some of the difficulties ambulance staff may experience when attempting to navigate how best to care for a patient.

Therefore, the process of deciding what is best for a person will involve a consideration of medical need. Murphy-Jones and Timmons (2016) explored the decision-making process of paramedics when deciding whether to convey to hospital or leave at home. Ambulance staff disclosed that patients' best interests were evaluated by considering the patient's current diagnosis and quality of life; the potential for alleviating or increasing psychological distress; the patient's wishes; pain management; and then weighing these up against the transport to hospital, moving the patient, possible exposure to infection, and possible legal consequences for making wrong decisions.

In weighing up whether to transport a person to hospital, consideration is given to family and carers, but also the views of other healthcare professionals. It might be the case that a physician discusses the current case via telephone with ambulance staff and is, therefore, unable to fully understand the dynamics of the situation. Advice given in such circumstances places a degree of responsibility on the staff at the scene to make the final choice.

There is also the influence of nursing staff who work within a care facility, or the reaction given to ambulance staff at hospital for conveying a patient. Jensen et al. (2013) highlighted several cultural and organisational barriers faced by ambulance clinicians, which may hinder interprofessional interactions when handing over a patient to another healthcare professional.

We may be requested to take a person we care for to hospital only to be greeted with a negative response, which impacts on the perception and competency of future care for the patient and family (Erbay, 2014). There is also a need to ensure, when consulting with the LPA, that their scope includes health and social care decisions, not just financial matters.

Waldrop et al. (2018) investigated how pre-hospital providers become mediators between ambulance services and emergency departments by managing tension, conflict and challenges in patient care. It is important that the processes for interprofessional working and collaboration are addressed to ensure safe treatment and transfer of vulnerable patients between facilities.

In terms of gaining consent, our first reference point should be the UK ambulance guidelines (JRCALC, 2019), whilst providing patients the opportunity to ask questions and seek clarity regarding any treatments and their outcomes (Riordan et al., 2015). There must not be any kind of coercion on the part of the family or ambulance staff. Consent must be voluntary, and patients should have the autonomy to withdraw consent at any time and change their mind. If consent is obtained under fear of harm or injury, intimidation, misrepresentation of information and facts, and misconception in the part of the patient and their family, then consent can be rendered invalid (Nijhawan et al., 2013).

To achieve meaningful and informed consent processes, it is imperative that ambulance clinicians fully understand the concepts behind informed consent. When discussing medical history with the patient, they may wish that their medical information remains a private matter and is not disclosed to a family member. It might be the case that the patient has a condition that not only affects them but also other family members, for example, genetic mutations.

Information can be disclosed to healthcare professionals when full disclosure has not occurred to all those who are affected. It is not reasonable that patients are always able to gain consent from family members for such information, as this would be impractical.

To achieve meaningful and informed consent processes, it is imperative that ambulance staff understand what health information sharing entails (Medical Research Council, 2007; Young, 2010).

A patient's understanding and perception of the risks of a medical intervention is dependent on a number of factors, for example, level of education, and is variable. Ambulance staff should provide information to patients that includes all potential side effects, but it would not be possible to provide a definitive list of side effects, thus undermining autonomy. In practice, when patients interact with a healthcare professional, they may choose to be selective in what type of information they provide.

In medical practice there are assumptions made about what a patient is consenting to, for example, if a patient consents to one treatment (which might also be connected to another intervention, e.g. cannula and drug), then they must have consented to both, which is not necessarily true.

The assumptions made with this type of thinking is that a process of implied consent, say holding an arm out to take a blood pressure, assumes that this type of consent covers all subsequent procedures. Gaining specific consent for specific medical interventions ensures that the process of gaining consent reaches beyond the interventions that you have provided details of (Kirk et al., 2017).

Summary

The *Mental Capacity Act* provides an overarching basis for ethical decision making in ambulance practice. We should ensure that in our interactions we can clearly assess capacity and fully understand the principles of autonomy, informed consent, and confidentiality. The tools and documents used to help advance treatments and care should be utilised at every opportunity, in particular advance care plans and best interest processes. We should consult patients at all times and those with LPA, in conjunction with other healthcare professionals responsible for the care of the patient, while maintaining dignity and privacy. We must consider our patients' cultural and religious beliefs and provide documentation of patients' wishes for medical care in the event of future incapacity. Ambulance clinicians, through a deep understanding of the ethical theories and issues, can facilitate the wishes of the person in end of life care and provide support for carers and family.

References

Alonso A, Dörr D and Szabo K (2017). Critical appraisal of advance directives given by patients with fatal acute stroke: an observational cohort study. *BMC Medical Ethics*, 18(1): 7.

Armitage E and Jones C (2017). Paramedic attitudes towards DNACPR orders. *Journal of Paramedic Practice*, 9(10): 445–452.

Avery G (2017). *An Introduction to Healthcare Ethics in Law and Ethics in Nursing and Healthcare* (2nd ed.). London: Sage, 23–26.

Beauchamp TL and Childress JF (2013). *Principles of Biomedical Ethics* (7th ed.). Oxford: Oxford University Press.

Bossaert L et al. (2015). European Resuscitation Council Guidelines for Resuscitation 2015: Section 11. The ethics of resuscitation and end-of-life decisions. *Resuscitation*, 95: 302–311.

Brady M (2013). A good death: key conceptual elements to end of life care. *Journal of Paramedic Practice*, 5(11): 624–630.

Brady M (2014). Challenges UK paramedics currently face in providing fully effective end-of-life care. *International Journal of Palliative Nursing*, 20(1): 37–44.

Brown EA (2014). Ethnic and cultural challenges at the end of life: setting the scene. *Journal of Renal Care*, 40: 2–5.

Caldwell G (2015). Full cardiopulmonary resuscitation should not be used for ordinary dying. *BMJ (Clinical Research Ed.)*, 351: h3769.

Choong KA (2015). Islam and palliative care. *Global Bioethics*, 26(1): 28–42.

Clarfield A et al. (2003). Ethical issues in end-of-life geriatric care: the approach of three monotheistic religions – Judaism, Catholicism, and Islam. *Journal of The American Geriatrics Society*, 51(8): 1149–1154.

Corrigan O (2003). Empty ethics: the problem with informed consent. *Sociology of Health and Illness*, 25(7): 768–792.

Delany C (2007). In private practice, informed consent is interpreted as providing explanations rather than offering choices: a qualitative study. *Australian Journal of Physiotherapy*, 53: 171–177.

Delany C (2008). Making a difference: incorporating theories of autonomy into models of informed consent. *Journal of Medical Ethics*, 34(9): e3.

Department of Health (2005). *Mental Capacity Act*. London, HMSO.

Detering K et al. (2010). The impact of advance care planning on end of life care in elderly patients: randomised controlled trial. BMJ *(Clinical Research Ed.)*, 340: c1345.

Erbay H (2014). Some ethical issues in prehospital emergency medicine. *Turkish Journal of Emergency Medicine*, 14(4): 193–198.

Evans C et al. (2017). Repeated emergency medical services use by older adults: analysis of a comprehensive statewide database. *Annals of Emergency Medicine*, 70(4): 506–515.

Evans N et al. (2012). A critical review of advance directives in Germany: attitudes, use and healthcare professionals' compliance. *Patient Education and Counseling*, 87(3): 277–288.

Ferri C and Jacob K (2017). Dementia in low-income and middle-income countries: different realities mandate tailored solutions. *Plos Medicine*, 14(3): e1002271.

Glick SM (2016). Jewish medical ethics. *The Israel Medical Association Journal: IMAJ*, 18(10): 577–580.

Greenberger C (2015). Enteral nutrition in end of life care: the Jewish Halachic ethics. *Nursing Ethics*, 22(4): 440–451.

HCPC (2014). *Standards of Proficiency*. London: Health and Care Professions Council.

HCPC (2016). *Standards of Conduct, Performance and Ethics*. London: Health and Care Professions Council.

Iserson KV (2006). Ethical principles – emergency medicine. *Emergency Medicine Clinics of North America*, 24(3): 513–545.

Jensen SM, Lippert A and Østergaard D (2013). Handover of patients: a topical review of ambulance crew to emergency department handover. *Acta Anaesthesiologica Scandinavica*, 57(8): 964–970.

Jotkowitz A and Zivotofsky A (2010). 'Love your neighbor like yourself': a Jewish ethical approach to the use of pain medication with potentially dangerous side effects. *Journal of Palliative Medicine*, 13(1): 67–71.

JRCALC and AACE (2019). *JRCALC Clinical Guidelines 2019*. Bridgwater: Class Professional Publishing.

Kant I (1996) *The Metaphysics of Morals (Cambridge Texts in the History of Philosophy)* (Gregor M, Ed.). Cambridge: Cambridge University Press.

Kinzbrunner BM (2004). Jewish medical ethics and end-of-life care. *Journal of Palliative Medicine*, 7(4): 558–573.

Kirk A (2018). Advanced care planning in end-of-life care: the key role of ambulance services. *Journal of Paramedic Practice*, 10(9): 1–4.

Kirk A et al. (2017). Paramedics and their role in end-of-life care: perceptions and confidence. *Journal of Paramedic Practice*, 9(2): 71–79.

Lambert S et al. (2017). Impact of informal caregiving on older adults' physical and mental health in low-income and middle-income countries: a cross-sectional, secondary analysis based on the WHO's study on global ageing and adult health (SAGE). *BMJ Open*, 7(11): e017236.

Leadership Alliance for the Care of Dying People (2014). *One chance to get it right: Improving people's experience of care in the last few days and hours of life*. Available at: https://www.gov.uk/government/uploads/system/uploads/attachment_data/file/323188/One_chance_to_get_it_right.pdf.

Leong L and Crawford G (2018). Residential aged care residents and components of end of life care in an Australian hospital. *BMC Palliative Care*, 17(1): 84.

Levi B and Green M (2010). Too soon to give up: re-examining the value of advance directives. *The American Journal of Bioethics: AJOB*, 10(4): 3–22.

Macnair T (1999). Medical ethics. *BMJ*, 319: S2–7214.

Maruthappu M, Sood H and Keogh B (2014). The NHS Five Year Forward View: transforming care. *The British Journal of General Practice: The Journal of the Royal College of General Practitioners*, 64(629): 635.

Mason E et al. (2016). Unscheduled care admissions at end-of-life – what are the patient characteristics? *Acute Medicine*, 15(2): 68–72.

Medical Research Council (2007). *The Use of Personal Health Information in Medical Research*. Medical Research Council, UK.

Moffat S et al. (2019). 'Do not attempt CPR' in the community: the experience of ambulance clinicians. *Journal of Paramedic Practice*, 11(5): 198–204.

Murphy-Jones G and Timmons S (2016). Paramedics' experiences of end-of-life care decision making with regard to nursing home residents: an exploration of influential issues and factors. *Emergency Medicine Journal: EMJ*, 33(10): 722–726.

National End of Life Care Programme (2017). *The Route to Success in end of life care— achieving quality in ambulance services.* 2012 [updated 2017] Available at: https://www.england.nhs.uk/improvement-hub/wp-content/uploads/sites/44/2017/11/End-of-Life-Care-Route-to-Success-ambulance-services.pdf.

Nijhawan L et al. (2013). Informed consent: issues and challenges. *Journal of Advanced Pharmaceutical Technology and Research*, 4(3): 134–140.

Ohr S, Jeong S and Saul P (2017). Cultural and religious beliefs and values, and their impact on preferences for end-of-life care among four ethnic groups of community-dwelling older persons. *Journal of Clinical Nursing*, 26(11/12): 1681–1689.

O'Neill O (2003). Some limits of informed consent. *Journal of Medical Ethics*, 29(1): 4–7.

Pecanac K et al. (2014). Respecting Choices® and advance directives in a diverse community. *Journal of Palliative Medicine*, 17(3): 282–287.

Qureshi A et al. (2013). Impact of advanced healthcare directives on treatment decisions by physicians in patients with acute stroke. *Critical Care Medicine*, 41(6): 1468–1475.

Rajagopal S et al. (2016). Characteristics of patients who are not resuscitated in out of hospital cardiac arrests and opportunities to improve community response to cardiac arrest. *Resuscitation*, 109: 110–115.

Ramasamy Venkatasalu M et al. (2018). Public, patient and carers' views on palliative and end-of-life care in India. *International Nursing Review*, 65(2): 292–301.

Riordan F et al. (2015). Patient and public attitudes towards informed consent models and levels of awareness of Electronic Health Records in the UK. *International Journal of Medical Informatics*, 84(4): 237–247.

Roache R (2014). Why is informed consent important? *Journal of Medical Ethics: Journal of the Institute of Medical Ethics*, 40(7): 435–436.

Sampson E et al. (2018). Living and dying with advanced dementia: a prospective cohort study of symptoms, service use and care at the end of life. *Palliative Medicine*, 32(3): 668–681.

Satyanarayana Rao KH (2008). Informed consent: an ethical obligation or legal compulsion? *Journal of Cutaneous and Aesthetic Surgery*, 1(1): 33–35.

Smythe A et al. (2017). A qualitative study investigating training requirements of nurses working with people with dementia in nursing homes. *Nurse Education Today*, 50: 119–123.

Steinberg A (2003). *Suffering in Encyclopedia of Jewish Medical Ethics*. Jerusalem: Feldheim Publishers.

Sutherland E et al. (2012). Clinical year in review III: asthma, chronic obstructive pulmonary disease, environmental and occupational lung disease, and ethics and end-of-life care. *Proceedings of the American Thoracic Society*, 9(4): 197–203.

Tirkkonen J et al. (2016). Ethically justified treatment limitations in emergency situations. *European Journal of Emergency Medicine: Official Journal of the European Society for Emergency Medicine*, 23(3): 214–218.

Tuckett AG (2012). The experience of lying in dementia care: a qualitative study. *Nursing Ethics*, 19(1): 7–20.

United Kingdom: Human Rights Act 1998 [United Kingdom of Great Britain and Northern Ireland], 9 November 1998. Available at: http://www.refworld.org/docid/3ae6b5a7a.html.

Upton, H. (2011). Moral theory and theorizing in health care ethics. *Ethical Theory and Moral Practice*, 14(4): 431–443.

van Wijmen et al. (2010). Advance directives in the Netherlands: an empirical contribution to the exploration of a cross-cultural perspective on advance directives. *Bioethics*, 24(3): 118–126.

Voss S et al. (2017). Home or hospital for people with dementia and one or more other multimorbidities: what is the potential to reduce avoidable emergency admissions? The HOMEWARD Project Protocol. *BMJ Open*, 7(4): e016651.

Waldrop DP (2014). Preparation for frontline end-of-life care: exploring the perspectives of paramedics and emergency medical technicians. *Journal of Palliative Medicine*, 17(3): 338–341.

Waldrop D (2015). Prehospital providers' perceptions of emergency calls near life's end. *American Journal of Hospice and Palliative Medicine*, 32(2): 198–204.

Waldrop D, McGinley J and Clemency B (2018). Mediating systems of care: emergency calls to long-term care facilities at life's end. *Journal of Palliative Medicine*, 21(7): 987–991.

Wendler D and Rid A (2011). Systematic review: the effect on surrogates of making treatment decisions for others. *Annals of Internal Medicine*, 154(5): 336–346.

Westra A, Willems D and Smit B (2009). Communicating with Muslim parents: 'The four principles' are not as culturally neutral as suggested. *European Journal of Pediatrics*, 168(11): 1383–1387.

Wiese C et al. (2012). Paramedics' end of life decision making in palliative emergencies. *Journal of Paramedic Practice*, 4(7): 413–419.

Yen Y et al. (2018). Association of advance directives completion with the utilization of life-sustaining treatments during the end-of-life care in older patients. *Journal of Pain And Symptom Management*, 55(2): 265–271.

Young R (2010). Informed consent and patient autonomy. In: *A Companion to Bioethics*. Oxford: Wiley-Blackwell.

Zieske M and Abbott J (2011). Ethics seminar: The hospice patient in the ED: an ethical approach to understanding barriers and improving care. *Academic Emergency Medicine: Official Journal of the Society for Academic Emergency Medicine*, 18(11): 1201–1207.

Chapter 8

Professional Resilience
Lindsay Hart

Introduction

While the role of the paramedic is forever evolving due to the growing diversity of the patient demographic and from the shift into delivering care in the community setting, the fundamental core elements of the job remain the same. The role of the paramedic is, first and foremost, to provide high-quality care and support to those who require their services. To be the clinician who is invited into a patient's home, often during desperate times, and entrusted to provide treatment and guidance to try to improve a situation, is an immense privilege.

The fast-paced, dynamic nature of paramedicine brings excitement and challenge, which may have drawn the individual to train as a paramedic in the first place. Both intrinsic and extrinsic motivators, such as the desire to 'save lives', 'help people', 'to have an exciting career' and to be 'part of an admired and trusted profession' have been identified as some of the motivational reasons to join the paramedic profession (Ross et al., 2016). The last motivator – 'to be part of an admired and trusted profession' – echoes results of studies on multiple occasions in multiple countries reporting paramedics to be one of the most trusted professions (Moloney and Batt, 2017). This accolade is a reflection of the high esteem that paramedics are held in by the general public across the globe.

While such favourable perceptions of the paramedic profession by the general population cannot be doubted, are we asking too much of paramedics to continuously perform in ever-changing and often distressing situations, shift after shift, without detriment to their wellbeing? Nationally, demand on the ambulance service is increasing by approximately 5.2% average annual growth since 2011/2012 (National Audit Office, 2017), and the scope of paramedic practice now requires paramedics to care for a wider complexity of patients in a more comprehensive manner (Brady, 2014). Research has identified that paramedics are at high risk of stress and burnout, with the paramedics themselves describing the fast pace and emotional intensity of the workload as particular stressors (Regehr and Millar, 2007).

While there will be other reasons why stress and burnout is prevalent in the profession, the inevitable exposure to death and dying can certainly be considered to be a potential stressor. The changing tides of the pre-hospital workload include patients who are receiving palliative care or who are approaching the end of their life, and as such, often present with differing psychological, social and spiritual needs (Brady, 2014). The preparedness and confidence that the paramedic feels in coping with these patients, and indeed their families, will vary from individual to individual. It is not just a simple case of providing treatment for end of life patients – there are other complexities involving legal and ethical concerns, communicating effectively and occasionally mediating within the family dynamic. Paramedics within the United Kingdom work within a set of guidelines and Trust-specific protocols. Confidence around the ability to work within these guidelines and protocols will depend upon the individual clinician, the knowledge and interpretation of these protocols, and how clearly and concisely they are written. The latter point can be seen as particularly important as it has been suggested that decision making in the pre-hospital environment may be difficult or problematic without clear directives (Waldrop et al., 2015), further adding to the anxieties felt by paramedics attending the end of life patient. Similarly, the confidence and conceptual knowledge that the paramedic possesses around end of life care will depend on the level and quality of education that they have received in the subject. Research by Rogers et al. (2015) concluded that while paramedics had some grasp of palliative care principles, these could be improved, with further inferences from a separate study suggesting the need for focusing upon the interrelationship between end of life and pre-hospital care through improved education and training (Waldrop et al., 2014). One of the strategy points identified by the Association of Ambulance Chief Executives (2014) is that there should be 'investment in regular education and training in end of life (care) for ambulance clinicians'. With an improved focus on education and training, perhaps some of the anxieties felt by the paramedic to cater for the complexities of end of life patients can be reduced or alleviated, thus moderating another area of stress that the paramedic faces.

However, as previously mentioned, factors affecting the paramedic attending an end of life patient are multifaceted and variable. The following chapter aims to consider some of the particular intricacies facing the paramedic by focusing on the following topics:

- Paramedic culture around death
- Conflict and the end of life patient
- Palliative care research and 'getting it right'
- Psychological demands of paramedic practice
- Professional resilience
- Detachment, compartmentalising and emotional blunting
- The use of humour.

Paramedic Culture Around Death

If asked, the majority of paramedics would probably state the ability to save lives as one of their drivers for undertaking the career that they have. To manage the end of life patient effectively requires a change in the mindset of these individuals. To move focus from saving a life to watching and allowing a patient to die is not easy, due in part to the instinctive reaction to intervene and provide aid to help and try to make the situation better. Practically, it may be seen by some paramedics as a challenge of their personal identity and a direct juxtaposition of what they are trained to do. Perhaps more emotionally challenging is the feeling of helplessness or even inadequacy in watching a patient die, especially when the death is distressing for the patient or the relatives.

Is it a failure for the patient to die? It has certainly been suggested that Western cultures may see death as a failure of medical science, rather than the natural end point to life (Chaturvedi et al., 2009). Perhaps then, the focal shift should be that the way the paramedic attended the scene, made the patient comfortable, and supported and counselled the relatives is actually the best outcome in terms of providing first class end of life care.

Conflict and the End of Life Patient

Guidance issued around caring for dying adults in the last days of their life (NICE, 2016) is directed at various healthcare professionals, including primary care clinicians. One element of this guidance is the importance of creating an individualised care plan, taking into account the dying person's wishes, personal care setting, preference for symptom management and any specified needs after death. While the existence of a care plan is vitally important for the patient in empowering them and involving them in their individual choices and preferences, paramedics can feel an overwhelming responsibility in attempting to honour these wishes. Evidence shows that families have reported calling for an emergency ambulance for the end of life patient for various reasons including falls, loss of consciousness, for an unplanned transfer to hospital when the patient deteriorates suddenly, or due to a reduction in the carers' ability to cope (Ingleton et al., 2009). How these specific situations are managed by the paramedic can influence not only where the patient will die, but also if the patient's end of life care choices are upheld (Waldrop et al., 2015).

Paramedics are invited into the homes of their patients and trusted to provide sound care and advice at a time when vulnerability and the emotional needs of those on scene may be at their highest (Moloney and Batt, 2017). End of life situations, in particular, may be emotionally charged situations that the paramedic is expected to effectively cope with. The emotions expressed by the patient, family or others at the scene may be varied and extreme, resulting in the need for the paramedic to dynamically adapt their communication and interpersonal skills. A type of witnessed reaction by family members following a death has been described as 'emotional desperation', with the family begging for medical intervention for their loved one (Waldrop et al., 2015). An example of such a case could manifest when the patient has a valid Do Not Attempt Cardiopulmonary Resuscitation (DNACPR) order, but when death occurs, the family call for an ambulance and implore the paramedic to intervene and provide treatment to try to resuscitate the patient. The stresses on the paramedic are great in this situation – they have a legal obligation to uphold the DNACPR and a moral obligation to the patient. Similar stresses occur in the opposite scenario when no legal documentation has been completed and as such the paramedic has a potential obligation to attempt cardiopulmonary resuscitation

(CPR), yet the family do not wish for this to happen and refuse to let the paramedic follow their protocols. Such intense emotions and the unrealistic demands of family members can make the environment unpredictable and the paramedic, whether working alone or as part of a crew, needs to have awareness of their own personal safety, especially in the unfamiliar and confined environment of the patient's home (Waldrop et al., 2015).

Advocacy, while described as a developing role for the paramedic (Moloney and Batt, 2017), is important throughout the patient journey, but arguably more so at the end of life when emotional and practical support may be desperately needed. The paramedic should aim to safeguard the rights of the patient, even if it conflicts with the views of the family (Moloney and Batt, 2017). However obvious this may seem in theory, becoming faced with these heightened states of distress or potentially even hostility from individuals within the patient's home may make it extremely difficult for the paramedic to become an effective advocate for the patient and their wishes. Such inconsistencies between the wishes of the patient and that of the relatives can lead to a stressful working environment, in which the paramedic has to manage not only the patient and their associated complexities, but also be aware of the needs of other individuals on scene. It may also be possible that the patient's relatives may be unaware of the wishes and desires of the individual or vice versa. There may be collusion, defined as information around the diagnosis, medical details or prognosis of the patient being not shared or even withheld between the individuals involved (Chaturvedi et al., 2009). As emergency responders, paramedics work in a dynamic environment, seeing a large number of patients and, as such, do not have the opportunity to build an ongoing relationship or develop a deep understanding of the relatives and their family dynamic. With this in mind, the first challenge for the paramedic will be to recognise the element of collusion and from there, manage communication and dialogue sensitively with either the patient or the relative to ensure that confidentiality is not breached.

Quite apart from the emotional and legal aspects discussed, the patient and their family will be unique in their cultural and spiritual needs. How these needs are addressed should be underpinned by communication that cultivates respect, support, concern and care. This is not just shown in a verbal context – gestures and attitudes will also have purpose (Chaturvedi et al., 2009). Guidance from the National Institute for Health and Care Excellence (NICE, 2011) recommends holistic assessments and considerations with regard to, among others, the spiritual and cultural needs of the patient. However, in terms of spiritual needs in particular, the Department of Health (DoH) found that a shift from perceived importance to practice was not always aligned (DoH, 2010). This, again, adds another layer to the complexity of the needs of the end of life patient that need to be addressed.

Each of these elements described singularly would be stressful for any clinician to deal with. When multiplied and set in the pre-hospital environment, it appears that the paramedic needs to be able to manage and adapt to the emotional demands of each situation (Christopher, 2006) before they even begin to consider the clinical aspects of managing a patient at the end of their life.

Palliative Care Research and 'Getting it Right'

The National End of Life Care Intelligence Network (2015) has produced data from two separate ambulance trusts within the United Kingdom. One of the considerations detailed by this research is that for ambulance staff who attend a patient at the end of their life, there may not be the key information regarding the patient's medical history or advance decisions to refuse cardiopulmonary resuscitation accessible. Certainly, it has been documented in qualitative interviews with emergency medical services (EMS) providers that missing documentation, such as DNACPR forms, has led to conflict with family members and even EMS colleagues around the decision to provide treatment (Waldrop et al., 2015).

An example of collaborative working among the differing agencies has been shown in the introduction of 'just in case' medications. These anticipatory medicines are available within the patient's home for acute symptom control. Obviously, the exacerbation of symptoms can occur at any time, day or night, and can require a prompt response. Before the introduction of these medications, depending on the availability or accessibility of specialist advice and certain medicines, the paramedics may have had little choice other than to convey the patient to an emergency department for symptom control. The impact of such conveyance on a patient who is already in pain or distressed should not be underestimated. It is without doubt a much better situation for all involved to be able to manage symptoms swiftly, with the patient comfortable in their own home.

As demonstrated in the previous section, the practical demands placed on the paramedic in managing the needs of the end of life patient can be complicated. However, the emotional demands can be just as, if not more, challenging. The emotional resilience of the paramedic is being constantly tested when they are, by the nature of their job, being exposed to traumatic scenes and death and dying on a frequent basis.

The aim of the next section of this chapter is to look at what can affect the paramedics' resilience and examine some of the coping strategies that are employed by the individual to deal with the emotional stresses of traumatic or emotive incidents. Whether or not these are effective or even healthy will depend on the individual and what strategies they choose to employ.

Consideration of the following elements of resilience will be discussed:

- Psychological demands of paramedic practice
- Professional resilience.

Further discussion centres on recognised coping mechanisms, such as:

- Detachment, compartmentalising and emotional blunting
- The use of humour.

Psychological Demands of Paramedic Practice

Research from the mental health charity MIND shows that emergency services personnel are more likely to experience a mental health problem than the general workforce, with 91% of ambulance personnel having experienced stress or poor mental health (MIND, 2015). The causes of mental health issues are very personal and individual and may occur acutely or in a more chronic and sustained way. Research shows that both acute and longstanding mental health can have physical implications, such as elevated cortisol levels, indicators of cardiovascular disease and poor sleep, and psychological impacts, for instance manifestations of depression, anxiety and post-traumatic stress disorder (PTSD) (Barbee et al., 2015).

PTSD, defined as an anxiety disorder that develops after exposure to a traumatic event, can manifest in a variety of ways. These can include memories of the event that can occur night or day and are so vivid that the individual feels that they are reliving the experience (Parkes and Prigerson, 2010). While the study into causative features of PTSD by Clohessy and Ehlers (1999) rated incidents involving children as the most stressful and among the most common incidents leading to intrusive memories, it has been conversely proposed that it is often the smaller, less sensational incidents that trigger an emotional response that leads to sustained effects on the individual (Regehr et al., 2002). Alternatively, it has been suggested that the cumulative effect of the exposure to distressing incidents and death depletes the emotional reserves of the paramedic and their ability to provide compassion. Compassion fatigue is documented as causing similar psychological distress to PTSD, characterised by a multitude of issues, such as depression, exhaustion and frustration, alongside negative emotions, including avoidance, fear and hyper-vigilance (Van Mol et al., 2015). Compassion fatigue has been explained as the expenditure of compassionate energy that outstrips the ability to recover from it (Boyle, 2011). While there is ongoing discussion around differences between compassion fatigue and burnout – the latter described as a work-related condition caused when stressful situations are endured (Montero-Marin et al., 2014) – both require the individual to develop coping mechanisms and, therefore, foster their own resilience.

Personal resilience is a fluid phenomenon and as such may not be as robust as needed, depending on other factors that the paramedic is coping with, either within the workplace or within their personal life. When faced with an emotive end of life patient scenario, for example, the paramedic may already be in an emotionally vulnerable state, especially if the incident is one that they can resonate with. There may be similarities with the patient scenario, for example, 'the incident is too close to home' – essentially the paramedic draws parallels with the patient, the scenario or the scene – or simply by over-sympathising or over-empathising with the relatives and, in effect, living their distress with them.

While it is indicated in literature that empathy can improve a variety of aspects of healthcare practice for both the patient and the clinician, it is suggested that valuable empathy can only be demonstrated by the clinician when they are in a positive frame of mind and without suffering from stress or burnout (Zenasni et al., 2012).

A challenge for the paramedic in this scenario will be to manage their emotions and to try to develop clinical empathy, thus recognising the feelings of patients (Zenasni et al., 2012) without becoming too emotionally involved and risking their own mental health. How this is achieved is complex, as Halpern (2003) suggests that emotions are typically outside the immediate control of most individuals, with empathy often being displayed instinctively (Adams, 2012).

When analysing the concept of emotional intelligence, which has been defined as combining emotions and their subdivisions – perceiving, using, understanding and managing emotions – with intelligence to help the individual to understand their social environment (Salovey and Grewal, 2005), it would appear that the fourth subdivision, managing (or regulating) emotion, links in with certain elements of clinical empathy. To regulate emotions requires the ability to alter an emotional response, with emotional management demanding the ability to evaluate the appropriateness of this response in different situations (Vandewaa et al., 2016). Managing their emotional response will help the paramedic to establish boundaries in their interaction with the patient scenario and their own vulnerability. Benefits of this are shown in data collected from the study into emotional intelligence by Wilson (2014), which found that healthcare workers who maintained these clear boundaries in their interaction with their patients reported that it enabled them to manage the emotional stress that they felt at work, whereas those who didn't discussed difficulty sleeping and intrusive thoughts when at home. The ability to develop and maintain these clear boundaries could both protect the paramedic's mental health and also become one of many coping strategies to enable longevity in their chosen career.

It is entirely reasonable, and indeed encouraged, that after a demanding or challenging incident, a call to check on the wellbeing of the paramedic takes place. However, these incidents may not be the calls that have the highest emotional impact on the member of staff (Regehr et al., 2002) and as such, it would be very difficult to ensure that support is offered in this way at all times. Emotional difficulties of paramedic practice do not only have an influence on the paramedic, but also on their families. The study by Regehr (2005) revealed that when interviewed, spouses of paramedics witnessed a variety of emotions such as anger, intolerance, nightmares, mood swings and withdrawal from the family group. Overprotection of children within the family group was also reported. Recognising these far-reaching consequences of the psychological difficulties associated with the job cannot be dismissed. However, there can still be reluctance from the paramedic in admitting that support is needed. Barriers in accessing help have included recognising the emotion within the individual themselves and being afraid of the stigma when revealing their thoughts to others (Halpern et al., 2014). With this is mind, developing an open culture within the ambulance service that encourages both self-awareness and empowerment in asking for help could prove beneficial for both paramedics and their loved ones.

Professional Resilience

Resilience can be defined as 'the interaction between the individual properties of the individual and the set of external conditions that allow the individual's adaptation or resistance to different forms of adversity at different points of life' (Lawn et al., 2011). It has been suggested that people are not born with a resilient trait, rather resilience is developed as a bank of strategies that a person builds through facing life's difficulties (Lawn et al., 2011). Certainly, findings from the research into the nature of resilience in paramedic practice by Clompus and Albarren (2016) appear to identify that challenging early life encounters equipped the paramedics with a degree of strength and emotional reserve that they utilised within their professional role.

How the individual develops their own resilience will be unique to them and as previously mentioned, resilience is not a stagnant feature. It may be strengthened or weakened depending on other stresses or strains, which are particular to the individual at that time in their life. There has been minimal research into how paramedics deal with the challenges of their role and how they become resilient to the demands of their profession (Clompus and Albarren, 2016). One suggestion to prepare future paramedics for these demands is to introduce the concept of resilience while students are in higher education to equip them with the emotional strength and endurance that is needed (McAllister and McKinnon, 2009). One of the ways of providing this could be through the use of reflective practice, as reflecting on both personal practice and learning from other practitioners has been suggested as a way to build resilience (McAllister and McKinnon, 2009).

Reflective practice is by no means a new phenomenon in healthcare, and students are often first introduced to this concept in university (Koshy et al., 2017). Questions that often linger following a challenging or distressing incident are 'Did I do everything that I could?' and 'What could I do better next time?' The questioning of the paramedic's own clinical competence may be mediated by the use of informal debriefing with colleagues, either in the ambulance or in the crew room, or by support from managers or team leaders. Using reflection and peer review can allow you to find areas for improvement and as such improve your skill as a clinician (Koshy et al., 2017).

Detachment, Compartmentalising and Emotional Blunting

It has been described in literature that to be able to effectively respond to the demands of the incident that they are called to, paramedics may utilise a degree of mental detachment or a compartmentalising of the situation to disassociate themselves from the emotiveness of the incident (Clompus and Albarren, 2016). Some paramedics can be described as task orientated or task driven, essentially modifying or eliminating sources of occupational stress through a series of actions required to successfully complete the desired task (LeBlanc et al., 2011). This focus on the task in hand has been reported by paramedics to help them cope with the emotional demands on scene by visualising the next practical step of the task, rather than being drawn into the reactions in the environment (Regehr et al., 2002). Indeed, evidence suggests that these task-orientated paramedics display lower anxiety responses in acutely stressful situations (LeBlanc et al., 2011).

When given that the paramedic has been called to help, often during a stressful or emotive time, this detachment could be viewed as a pragmatic solution to the situation that they are faced with. However, this strategy is not without limitations.

Certain scenarios, such as trauma, often require a more task-orientated approach, which can allow a certain amount of detachment from the patient. In comparison, scenarios such as palliative and end of life care demand a greater amount of caring skills and emotional labour, meaning that this strategy may be more problematic (Clompus and Albarren, 2016). Emotional detachment can also potentially encroach into the personal life of the paramedic, with regards to being able to move to emotional openness, thus affecting relationships (Regehr et al., 2002).

The Use of Humour

Black humour, or gallows humour as it is also referred to, can be roughly defined as using humour in response to a situation that is serious or traumatic. Humour has long been recognised as a strategy for dealing with the demands of the paramedic role, with Palmer (1983) describing that humour may be used by paramedics as an escape or as a safety valve. This view is essentially echoed in later literature, which suggests that black humour can be used as a valuable defence mechanism, with the ability of utilising laughter as a means of physiological and psychological stress relief (Rowe and Regehr, 2010).

Humour within the ambulance service (and similarly, the police force) has been described as a 'mutually acceptable but culturally defined joke book designed for different occupations' (Charman, 2013). One of the functions of humour is to encourage group cohesion and camaraderie (Clompus and Albarren, 2016). Paramedics have been described in literature as a 'cohesive and insular group who prefer the company of other frontline personnel' (Halpern et al., 2009). This bond can be assumed to exist, in part, in order to share and understand the lived experiences of colleagues, with camaraderie within the group serving a deeper purpose in creating a support network, both within the profession and extending out to other colleagues in other frontline emergency services. Interestingly, social identity theory proposes that the individual's self-concept develops as a member of a particular social group (Rowe and Regehr, 2010). This group cohesion and camaraderie within the paramedic profession serves as a support system in itself, thus evidenced in an interview quoted in the study by Halpern et al. (2009), with one ambulance clinician stating that an incident early on in their career had caused significant distress as they had not yet formed a support network within the workplace.

It has been suggested that the use of humour as a mechanism for coping is vital for emergency personnel (Rowe and Regehr, 2010). The brief distraction that humour allows can shift the focus from the distress of the incident and enable the individual to regather their personal reserves and create an emotional barrier from a cognitive coping perspective (Rowe and Regehr, 2010). However, for the use of humour to exist in this fashion requires the paramedic to employ their professionalism. By its nature, the use of black humour can be interpreted differently by persons outside of the profession. The routine terminology used in relation to an upsetting situation could certainly be viewed as inappropriate or highly offensive by the lay person. Timing of the use of humour must be so that it is not utilised in front of the patient or their family (Rowe and Regehr, 2010). Similarly, boundaries exist within the profession as to the inclusion of the types of humour that can be used. Professionals may sanction their own conduct, but censorship as a group also exists to avoid the risk of causing offence (Scott, 2007). Usually, certain categories of patients would be seen as inappropriate to include in joking and humour. The context in which black humour is employed requires consideration too. The use of this coping mechanism should not be a disrespectful act by the paramedic. When humour involves negativity in a manner to dehumanise or devalue the patient, the individual's capacity to provide compassionate, high-level care could be questioned (Rowe and Regehr, 2010).

While the use of humour appears to be an important coping strategy, it has been suggested that the use of humour may only mask the effects of traumatic experiences (Charman, 2013). Therefore, it may be suggested that while humour and the other coping methods discussed may seem to help, each will have individual limitations, which should be recognised and therefore utilised as part of a more comprehensive approach, rather than relied upon in isolation.

Conclusion

When considering the increase in the ageing population, it is entirely reasonable to expect the paramedic profession to become more involved in palliative and end of life care. However, there are numerous challenges associated with this – training and education should enable the paramedic to have confidence in the levels of care that they can provide to the patient and their family and should encompass not only protocols, but also focus upon communication in end of life scenarios with an awareness of how to cope with challenges in adhering to the patients' wishes in the pre-hospital setting.

It is evident that the dynamic and often distressing nature of paramedicine is such that it can lead to significant levels of mental health conditions within the profession. Dealing with death is an inevitable part of practice, but the individual must be aware of the importance of building resilience and developing coping strategies to enable them to remain healthy in such a demanding role. The support of colleagues and more formal mechanisms, such as counselling, are invaluable. The same can be said of other coping mechanisms that have been discussed. It must, however, be recognised that these coping strategies have limitations associated with them and for a more comprehensive safeguard, the paramedic should be supported in taking ownership of their mental health and be reassured and actively encouraged to seek help to ensure both wellbeing and longevity in their chosen profession.

Case Studies

 Case Study 1

You and your paramedic crewmate are called to attend a 58-year-old man, Alan, who is known to have terminal lung cancer. He has been steadily deteriorating over the past few weeks and up until now, Sue, his wife, has been coping with his care. You are called today as the patient has slipped from bed and Sue requires help to get him back into bed. After doing so, Sue breaks down in tears and states that she can no longer cope with Alan and wants him to go into hospital so that she can have a break. Alan is worried for Sue's mental and physical health and agrees with Sue that he should go to the emergency department.

- How do you support both Sue and Alan?
- Can you suggest a more suitable solution than the emergency department?

✳ Case Study 2

You are working as a single responder on a car. You receive a 999 call to a 62-year-old woman, Molly, who is a known end of life patient. Molly has a valid DNACPR, which is handed to you on your arrival. It is clear that Molly has just gone into cardiac arrest and her daughter, Lucy, is hysterical and demanding that you intervene and perform CPR. Lucy will not listen to reason and starts to shout.

- How will you manage this situation?

✳ Case Study 3

While on shift with a paramedic crewmate Sam, you are called to an 80-year-old woman, Olive. Olive is a known palliative care patient and has been found dead in her bed by her 15-year-old grandson, Mark. Mark is understandably very distressed and your colleague deals with Mark while you complete relevant paperwork for Olive. The next time you work with Sam he is quiet and withdrawn. He confides in you that he is still troubled by the incident and isn't sleeping well. He identifies with Mark, as Sam had a similar experience with finding his aunt dead.

- What are your thoughts about what Sam says to you?
- What practical advice can you offer him?

Case Study 4

You are a paramedic working with a crewmate and are called to attend an 82-year-old man, Brian, who has severe shortness of breath. Brian has COPD and has had a chest infection, which he has not sought medical attention for. His daughter and son-in-law, Andrea and Paul are on scene. There is no DNACPR for Brian. While you are providing initial treatment, Brian goes into cardiac arrest. Both Andrea and Paul are adamant that you should not provide treatment as this is 'not what he would have wanted'.

- What are the legal and ethical considerations in this case?
- How will you manage this situation?

References

Adams R (2012). Clinical empathy: a discussion on its benefits for practitioners, students of medicine and patients. *Journal of Herbal Medicine*, 2(2): 52–57.

Association of Ambulance Chief Executives (2014). *Future National Clinical Priorities for Ambulance Services in England National Ambulance Service Medical Directors (NASMeD)*. Available at: https://aace.org.uk/wp-content/uploads/2014/05/Future-national-clinical-priorities-for-ambulance-services-in-England-FINAL-2.pdf.

Barbee A et al. (2015). EMS perspectives on coping with child death in an out-of-hospital setting. *Journal of Loss and Trauma*, 21(6): 455–470.

Boyle D (2011). Countering compassion fatigue: a requisite nursing agenda. *The Online Journal of Issues in Nursing*, 16(1): 2.

Brady M (2014). Challenges UK paramedics currently face in providing fully effective end-of-life care. *International Journal of Palliative Nursing*, 20(1): 37–43.

Charman S (2013). The role of humour in relationships between police officers and ambulance staff. *International Journal of Sociology and Social Policy*, 33: 152–166.

Chaturvedi S, Loiselle C and Chandra P (2009). Communication with relatives and collusion in palliative care: a cross-cultural perspective. *Indian Journal of Palliative Care*, 15(1): 2–9.

Christopher S (2006). *Dealing with Death and Dying: A Paramedic's Perspective*. Available at: https://www.researchgate.net/profile/Sarah_Christopher/publication/281447771_Dealing_with_death_and_dying_a_paramedic%27s_perspective/links/55e80e0a08aeb6516262f458/Dealing-with-death-and-dying-a-paramedics-perspective.pdf.

Clohessy S and Ehlers A (1999). PTSD symptoms, response to intrusive memories and coping in ambulance service workers. *British Journal of Clinical Psychology*, 38: 260.

Clompus S and Albarren J (2016). Exploring the nature of resilience in paramedic practice: a psycho-social study. *International Emergency Nursing*, 28: 1–7.

Department of Health (2010). *Spiritual Care at the End of Life*. University of Hull. Available at: https://www.gov.uk/government/uploads/system/uploads/attachment_data/file/215798/dh_123804.pdf.

Halpern J (2003). What is clinical empathy? *Journal of General Internal Medicine*, 18(8): 670–674.

Halpern J et al. (2009) What makes an incident critical for ambulance workers? Emotional outcome and implications for intervention. *Work and Stress*, 23(2): 173-189.

Halpern J et al. (2014). Downtime after critical incidents in emergency medical technicians/paramedics. *Biomed Research International*. Available at: https://www.ncbi.nlm.nih.gov/pmc/articles/PMC4024400/.

Ingleton C et al. (2009). Barriers to achieving care at home at the end of life: transferring patients between care settings using patient transport services. *Palliative Medicine*, 23(8): 725–726.

Koshy K et al. (2017). Reflective practice in health care and how to reflect effectively. *International Journal of Surgery: Oncology*, 2(6): e20.

Lawn S et al. (2011). 'I just saw it as something that would pull you down, rather than lift you up': resilience in never-smokers with mental illness. *Health Education Research*, 26(1): 26–38.

LeBlanc V et al. (2011), The association between posttraumatic stress, coping and acute stress responses in paramedics. *Traumatology*, 17(4): 10–16.

McAllister M and McKinnon M (2009). The importance of teaching and learning resilience in the health disciplines: a critical review of the literature. *Nurse Education Today*, 29(4): 371–379.

MIND (2015). *Ambulance – How to Manage Your Mental Wellbeing*. Available at: http://www.mind.org.uk/information-support/ambulance/mental-wellbeing-ambulance/#.Wb5qLMiGPIU.

Moloney B and Batt A (2017). The Paramedic as a Patient Advocate. *Canadian Paramedicine*, 38: 16–18.

Montero-Marin J et al. (2014). Coping with stress and types of burnout: explanatory power of different coping strategies. *PLOS ONE*. Available at: http://journals.plos.org/plosone/article?id=10.1371/journal.pone.0089090#s1.

National Audit Office (2017). *NHS Ambulance Services*. Available at: https://www.nao.org.uk/wp-content/uploads/2017/01/NHS-Ambulance-Services.pdf.

National End of Life Care Intelligence Network (2015). *Ambulance Data Project for End of Life Care*. London: Public Health England.

National Institute for Health and Care Excellence (2011). *End of Life Care for Adults*. Available at: https://www.nice.org.uk/guidance/qs13.

National Institute for Health and Care Excellence (2016). *Care of Dying Adults in the Last Days of Life*. Available at: https://www.nice.org.uk/guidance/ng31.

Palmer C (1983). A note about paramedic's strategies for dealing with death and dying. *Journal of Occupational Psychology*, 56: 83–86.

Parkes C and Prigerson H (2010). *Bereavement: Studies of Grief in Adult Life* (4th ed.). London: Routledge.

Regehr C (2005). Bringing the trauma home: spouses of paramedics. *Journal of Loss and Trauma*, 1: 105–107.

Regehr C, Goldberg G and Hughes J (2002). Exposure to human tragedy, empathy and trauma in ambulance paramedics. *American Journal of Orthopsychiatry*, 72(4): 505–513.

Regehr C and Millar D (2007), Situation critical: high demand, low control and low support in paramedic organizations. *Traumatology*, 13(1): 49–58.

Rogers I et al. (2015). Paramedics' perceptions and educational needs with respect to palliative care. *Australasian Journal of Paramedicine*, 12(5): 1–7.

Ross L, Hannah J and Huizen P (2016). What motivates students to pursue a career in paramedicine? *Australasian Journal of Paramedicine*, 13(1): 4.

Rowe A and Regehr C (2010). Whatever gets you through today: an examination of cynical humour among emergency service professionals. *Journal of Loss and Trauma*, 15: 448–464.

Salovey P and Grewal D (2005). The Science of Emotional Intelligence. *Current Directions in Psychological Science*, 14(6): 281–285.

Scott T (2007). Expressions of humour by emergency personnel involved in sudden death work. *Mortality*, 12(4): 350–364.

Vandewaa E, Turnipseed D and Cain G (2016). Panacea or placebo? An evaluation of the value of emotional intelligence in healthcare workers. *Journal of Health and Human Services Administration*, 38(4): 438–477.

Van Mol M et al. (2015). The prevalence of compassion fatigue and burnout among healthcare professionals in intensive care units: a systematic review. *PLoS One*, 10(8): e0136955.

Waldrop D et al. (2014). Preparation for frontline end-of-life care: exploring the perspectives of paramedics and emergency medical technicians. *Journal of Palliative Medicine*, 17(3): 338–341.

Waldrop D et al. (2015). 'We are strangers walking into their life changing event': how prehospital providers manage emergency calls at the end of life. *Journal of Pain and Symptom Management*, 50(3): 328–334.

Wilson J (2014). The awareness of emotional intelligence by nurses and support workers in an acute hospital setting. *Journal of Health Sciences*, 2(9): 458–464.

Zenasni F et al. (2012). Burnout and empathy in primary care: three hypotheses. *The British Journal of General Practice*, 62(600): 346–347.

| Chapter 9 | **The Paramedic as an End of Life Specialist**
Kath Jennings |

Introduction

This chapter aims to orientate the paramedic towards a deeper awareness of the circumstances around attending patients in receipt of palliative care and care for patients at the end of their life. While palliative care may be relevant to all healthcare professionals, it is the extended role of the paramedic as specialist practitioner in this field that will be considered here, including clinical decision making at the end of life. Case studies will be used to illustrate two scenarios followed by discussion using related evidence. There will be acknowledgement of the developing complexity of the paramedic role over time and identification of selected national and international research. The chapter ends with a reminder of the positive impact paramedics can have on palliative and dying patients drawing upon their expertise.

As a starting point, paramedics may look to the hospice movement, which provided great leaps forward in the understanding of holistic care for the dying and in reshaping understanding of the celebration of living as well as the preparation for death. Paramedics may learn much from the hospice movement, detailed elsewhere in this book, from physical symptom control to careful and thoughtful management of the environment when called to patients receiving palliative care. The terms 'palliative care' and 'end of life care' have sometimes mistakenly been used interchangeably reflecting limited understanding of both the stages of illness and of the philosophy of care. Definitions of these terms have appeared elsewhere in this book, yet the idea of the paramedic as an end of life specialist is a developmental goal for the paramedic profession as a whole. By increasing knowledge and understanding of incurable illness and the dying process, and implementing truly patient-led care, paramedics may not only effectively and compassionately manage patient care, but become palliative and end of life specialists.

Historically only cancer patients were understood to receive and benefit from palliative services, but awareness of palliative and end of life care among paramedics and other emergency care providers has grown as the number of people dying later in life with a long-term condition continues to increase. More than 15 million people in England have a long-term condition, defined as 'a health problem that can't be cured but can be controlled by medication or other therapies' (Department of Health, 2015), and the number of people living with three or more long-term conditions was predicted to rise to 2.9 million in 2018 (The Kings Fund, 2017). This phenomenon has not happened at any previous time in history and its uniqueness both contributes to the increasing workload of ambulance services and provides paramedics with an opportunity to develop knowledge, skills and attitudes regarding a growing group of the population. The causes of sudden unexpected death, such as cardiovascular disease and trauma, prevalent in the last third of the twentieth century, are being replaced by the more predictable decline in health to death, thus making possible the planning for death by individuals living with disease.

The Extended Role of Paramedics in the Care of Palliative and Dying Patients

There is a suggestion that the failed resuscitation of anyone nearly or newly dead leads to negative feelings or feelings of failure in paramedics (Brady, 2012). This may be due to the historical education and training of paramedics, which focused on the biomedical model of treatment and excluded the psychological, sociological or even spiritual impact of illness as experienced by patients. The cultural identity of paramedics as life savers has been reinforced by their portrayal in popular TV programmes. Yet for paramedics, palliative and end of life care has in common with other patient care episodes the careful and thorough assessment of the scene, the patient and the environment. And while paramedics may not be able to cure underlying disease, they have become experts at patient assessment and symptom control and management. In this way patients in receipt of palliative care and patients at the end of their lives can expect expert care from paramedics, and paramedics can aspire to become as confident in this area as they have become in the assessment and management of many other patient presentations.

Paramedics should be aware that a palliative care pathway may be in place up to two years before death. The call to a patient in receipt of palliative care therefore is not necessarily a call to a dying patient; but it might be. Paramedics preparing themselves en route to a patient in receipt of palliative care should be ready to meet with one of a range of presentations reflecting the different trajectories expected in the advancement of the patient's underlying condition. Existing literature identifies different trajectories of declining health and death (O'Connor, 2018). It is acknowledged that cancer patients in receipt of palliative care follow a fairly predictable decline in health, characterised by an increase in symptoms of pain, breathlessness, reduced appetite, increased nausea and reduced functional ability. Much less predictable in nature is the decline and death of a patient experiencing organ failure following long-term illness (congestive obstructive pulmonary disease, congestive heart failure, liver or kidney failure). These patients have periods of stability and periods of exacerbation of symptoms. With each exacerbation there will be a decline in overall health compared to prior to the episode and the disease trajectory will follow a decline punctuated by severe and sometimes violent illness. Dementia patients in receipt of palliative care may have little functional ability, experience symptoms atypically and have an overall steady decline (O'Connor, 2018).

While attending to a palliative care patient the paramedic will need to appreciate the philosophy of palliative care as an affirmation of life. The goal of the paramedic therefore is the improvement in the quality of life for the patient. Almost all patients in receipt of palliative care will have sufficient understanding of their condition to know that a cure is not being sought. In this way communication between paramedics and patients and their carers can be facilitated by paramedics adopting an open and truthful approach. It is the task for paramedics to integrate the principles of palliative care into emergency care practice. Open communication greatly facilitates this task. One key principle is that of person-centred care as a way of handing power back to the patient, who is seen as having a more active role to play in their own destiny. Practitioners and carers are encouraged to work with the patient in order to determine what kind of care and care environment should be selected. This can also include prior consideration being given to the playing of music, persons present or to be contacted. Pope (2012) describes the dimensions of person-centred care as:

- Listening to patients

- Treating patients as individuals

- Understanding patients' rights and values

- Respecting dignity and confidentiality

- Empowering individuals and encouraging autonomy

- Building mutual trust and understanding.

The paramedic as expert in palliative and end of life care will know that palliative care may be given in hospice or home. Some literature even identifies palliative care services being given to homeless people on the streets (O'Connor, 2018). Hospice attendance may be for respite only and may be admission or day attendance. Where palliative and end of life care has been planned and agreed in partnership between the patient, family and healthcare providers, the decision-making burden on immediate care providers such as paramedics is greatly relieved.

✵ Case Study 1

Emma was the paramedic who responded to a call to Jan. Jan had been receiving hospice care for the previous three days and earlier, on the morning of the 999 call, was transferred home to fulfil her wish to die at home. Later that evening Jan had become very distressed and her family (daughter, son-in-law and two granddaughters) had become very upset and concerned about Jan's levels of pain and comfort. On her arrival, Emma had ascertained that there was a care plan in place for this phase of Jan's life and death, which involved a palliative care nurse being in attendance, but there was as yet no nurse on scene. Rather than call the nurse Jan's daughter had called 999, because in that moment she did not know what else to do. Emma assessed Jan for any imminent threat to her life. She and her crewmate found that Jan's position in the bed was impeding her comfort and so they placed her on her side in the recovery position. Emma then reassured Jan and her family that she would make Jan more comfortable. She telephoned the palliative care nurse for advice and, since Jan's care plan included the administration of morphine, Emma was able to administer the drug and its sedative effect appeared to reduce Jan's discomfort. Emma considered administering oxygen and was careful to include this consideration in her telephone consultation with the expert palliative care nurse. During the episode of care, Jan had been incontinent of faeces. Emma and her crew mate were able to clean Jan and to change her clothing and bed linen. They washed her hands and face with warm water, soap and a flannel, and asked Jan's daughter to brush her hair how she would like it. When Jan was clean and comfortable the rest of her family entered the room and sat with her until she died. Now sitting in another room in the house, Emma and her crewmate also telephoned other family members, which was in the plan. She then telephoned the on-call hospice doctor to inform them of the actions taken and for any further advice pending the arrival of the nurse. Once the palliative care nurse arrived, Emma and her crew mate said goodbye to Jan and her family and left full documentation of their actions.

Discussion of Case Study 1

In this case study, Emma as a paramedic utilised a range of well-practiced and honed skills. First, she and her crew mate introduced a calm atmosphere to a previously highly charged scene; they then offered reassurance to a distressed family. Adapting skills originally learned for life support, Emma and her crew mate immediately tended to one element of the patient's presenting complaint. Using excellent communication skills, she was able to gather a further history and establish the existence of a care plan, and by effectively mobilising input from other experts involved in the patient's care, Emma was able to ensure correct treatment was delivered to manage the patient's symptoms. The crew were on scene for two and a half hours. They were able to effectively engage with Jan and her family, to have an extremely positive impact on the dying phase of Jan's life, and to effectively disengage, as they had done many times before. They were applying their knowledge and skills to end of life care resulting in the patient's needs and wishes being met. It is possible to see how Pope's dimensions of person-centred care have been played out.

The prevalence of pain as a significant feature of the end of life is often a reason for the making of an emergency call for help. Paramedics can utilise the World Health Organization's stepwise approach to pain management, discussed elsewhere in the book. The Association of Ambulance Chief Executives and Joint Royal Colleges Ambulance Liaison Committee's *Clinical Practice Guidelines* provide recommended dosages for the management of pain in the dying patient (JRCALC, 2019). Administration of opiates, as in Case Study 1, should follow this guidance in the absence of the patient's own personal medical plan being to hand. Further to this there may also be 'just in case' medication prescribed for the patient, which the paramedic can administer. Collaboration with a wider team is key to serving the patient's best interests, and in the absence of direct communication with the patient's team the paramedic can access a clinical hub for further input. Paramedics attending all patients must be aware of the limitations of their scope of practice and of any relevant patient-specific protocol (written, up-to-date treatment, which is administered to an individual outside of usual guidelines), or patient group directive (written, up-to-date treatment, which is administered to an identified group of patients outside of usual guidelines). There should be a good understanding of drug actions and the risks of administering them to the palliative patient for the management of symptoms. As well as pain management, consideration should be given to airway management, comfort, and to nausea and vomiting (JRCALC, 2019). This should be read alongside the full guidelines for the management of end of life care (JRCALC, 2019).

Paramedics and Clinical Decision Making at the End of Life

At the end of life, the intensifying need for care for the dying patient can cause significant distress for care givers and families. Furthermore, the presentation or exacerbation of unexpected symptoms can leave care givers feeling powerless or unable to express themselves normally. Paramedics are called when carers do not know what to do next when caring for their dying loved ones at home or in a care facility. A sudden deterioration or exacerbation may lead to a 999 call where on the arrival of the emergency crew there may be an expectation, realistic or otherwise, that intervention can lead to improvement in the dying person. It can be useful for paramedics to be mindful that how well they manage their response to calls to patients at the end of life determines how and where people will die. It may be a heavy responsibility to countenance that paramedic decision making may be the determining factor in whether or not a patient's end of life choice is upheld. Paramedics may feel an inherent contradiction in attending a patient at the end of their life regarding the paramedic's cultural identity as life saver as opposed to facilitator of death. The commencement of resuscitation is thought to be a safe and natural position for paramedics particularly when there may be a demand to 'do something'. Remaining focused on enabling a person to achieve care according to their needs and wishes (JRCALC, 2019) may provide a countervailing energy. By considering a 'good death' paramedics may enable for the dying person dignity, respect, familiarity of environment and faces, calmness and painlessness.

One definition of effective decision making is the selection of a course of action based upon its merits following due consideration of alternatives (Cork and Brady, 2019). This method follows a hypothetic deductive model of decision making utilised by paramedics, where it is necessary to collect information, to consider a range of alternatives and then to act to implement a decision. With knowledge of disease and deterioration trajectories and with experience, an attending paramedic can come to expect certain responses. A danger facing inexperienced paramedics when called to a patient at the end of their life is to consider that the only decisions to make are either to transport or not to transport to hospital, or to resuscitate or not. Paramedics should be guided by the JRCALC guideline for end of life care (JRCALC, 2019) to establish the appropriate care pathway with a view to facilitating any advance decision making that may have occurred. This practice is further supported by the Health and Care Professions Council Standards of conduct, ethics and performance, particularly regarding making informed and reasonable decisions by taking advice and support (Health and Care Professions Council, 2016). This is reinforced by taking a team-working and a shared decision-making approach. Effective management of patients at the end of life with regard to their holistic needs is facilitated by teamwork and by adopting an interdisciplinary approach. When arriving on scene, while there is some division of labour between the emergency crew, they essentially belong only to one discipline, which is that of pre-hospital or out-of-hospital care. They are disadvantaged because they have no prior relationship with the patient and have a lot of information to gather in a relatively short time. Early on in responding to the call, paramedics should remember that input from others involved in the patient's care will help to create order and put in place some of the steps that may have been identified in an advance care plan. This might involve telephoning the patient's GP or palliative care nurse for advice or guidance. There may be a spiritual leader to contact and invite to the scene, children to say goodbye to or pets to include for comfort, or selected music to play. All individuals connected with the patient at the end of their life constitute members of this interdisciplinary team, each having a role of equal importance in the eyes of the dying patient. For paramedics, developing an understanding of teamwork and accessing the wider team involved in the patient's care up to that point will inform and enhance their decision making. Further evidence available to facilitate decision making may be written and dated and signed by the patient or their lasting power of attorney.

In cases where little or no forward planning has taken place, paramedics attending a patient at the end of their life may have to undertake rapid and simultaneous assessments of the patient, their family or carers and of the environment. Assessment of the patient involves the medical presentation of the chief presenting complaint and its recent development; the taking and recording of vital signs, level of consciousness, stated pain or response to painful stimulus. The history taking will include the patient's diagnosis, prognosis and comorbidities. Assessment of the family or carers includes observing and judging family dynamics, identification of a spokesperson (lasting power of attorney or otherwise), the presence or absence of an advance directive, actual levels of emotional distress as well as potential levels of distress with arrival of additional family members. This overlaps with environmental assessment, which paramedics have to rapidly identify as potentially convivial or hazardous. Research by Waldrop et al. (2015) showed that paramedics stated that they could assess family and environmental dynamics in just five seconds and that the results of their assessment influenced their approach to the call. This in turn had an influence on where the patient died irrespective of their previously stated wishes, which may have been to die at home. Further complexities to the assessment and management of a patient at the end of their life in the absence of forward planning is that where resuscitation is attempted, paramedics must consider whether or not to involve family members or principal carers as witnesses to the resuscitation in order to demonstrate that everything that could possibly be done was done.

🩺 Case Study 2

Mo was the paramedic first responder to John. John had been diagnosed with lung cancer two years earlier, had become emaciated over the two years since diagnosis, and had recently experienced a marked decline in health. He was moved by his family (wife and son) into a downstairs room to ease mobility around the house and had aids in place for assisting his daily needs. He had in the last 12 hours been complaining of sweating excessively and breathlessness, so believing himself to have an infection had gone to bed early on the night that Mo attended. At 03.00 he was heard falling to the floor and on Mo's arrival John was unresponsive and was not breathing. Mo swiftly established cardiac arrest but observing the emaciated condition of John questioned his family further regarding John's recent and past medical history. Mo determined that John's diagnosis was two years earlier, that the prognosis was terminal and that no treatment interventions had been undertaken for months. Despite calling 999 on hearing the fall, when John's family realised he was in cardiac arrest, they requested that under the circumstances Mo did not commence a resuscitation attempt for John. When asked to supply a written Do Not Attempt Cardiopulmonary Resuscitation order, the family stated that they did not have one. Mo liaised with the family and between them they agreed that resuscitation would be futile.

Then an ambulance crew arrived. Despite Mo being senior clinician on scene, the ambulance crew questioned his decision not to resuscitate, and did so vocally and in front of John's family. This cast doubt in their minds over the decision they had reached regarding John's best interests, and they became distressed that enough was not being done for him. John's son then demanded loudly that everything should be done to try to save him, to give him more time. The crew began cardiopulmonary resuscitation and transported John to the nearest hospital where he was pronounced dead in the emergency department soon after arriving. His distressed family were transported in Mo's car driven by a junior crew member.

Discussion of Case Study 2

It is clear to see that Pope's dimensions of person-centred care were missing from the management of this patient. The non-existence of a clear plan hampered the emergency crew's collective ability to listen to wishes, to treat John as an individual and to understand and represent his rights and values. But it was the vocal disagreement among the emergency crew and paramedic that failed to build trust and understanding with John's family and eroded confidence. Paramedics must assess the knowledge and expectations held by family or care givers regarding any resuscitation attempt and to explain the limitations of intervention at the end of life. This knowledge will be otherwise unknown to the paramedic attending, impacting negatively upon their own confidence to 'promote the best interests of patients and their care givers' (Health and Care Professions Council, 2016).

The experience of the paramedic in the second case study is reflected by Murphy-Jones and Timmons (2016) in their research into paramedic decision making regarding the transport of patients at the end of their life from nursing home to emergency department. They found that the absence of advance decision making by patients and their carers or loved ones was a barrier to paramedic decision making and lead to uncertainty among the paramedic participants. Conflict is another barrier to decision making. Conflict can arise in the absence of legal order to not commence resuscitation where emergency responders feel duty bound to attempt to resuscitate the near death or deceased patient. Conflict may also arise even when there is a legal order in place not to resuscitate but family members or carers demand that 'something must be done'. While paramedics are ethically and legally bound to honour the patient's autonomy while capacity was held to complete the legal order, they may succumb to immense pressure to commence resuscitation and opt for a utilitarian ethical position of satisfying the greatest good for the greatest number, even if that position opposes the patient's wishes.

The Changing Education Requirements of Paramedics for Effective Palliative Care and the Impact of Research

It is essential that paramedic expertise is developed in the area of palliative and end of life care. When seen in the context of the development of paramedic education and practice over the past 50 years, paramedics have moved from being stretcher bearers in the field and street to expertly reversing threats to life; from transportation to triage, assessment, treatment, referral or discharge from care. Developments in pre-hospital cardiac and trauma care together with the reorganisation of services have led to increasing survival rates in these patient groups. Elsewhere improvements to the pre-hospital recognition and management of sepsis continue to drive research and reduce mortality from it.

There have been two periods of ground-breaking change in the development of paramedic practice and education in the last half century. First, the Miller reports of the mid 1960s looked critically at the trauma and transport focus of the post-war era and lead to the requirement of a first aid certificate and driving qualification for ambulance personnel. This evolved over the following decades into the Institute for Healthcare Development (IHCD) ambulance aid and ambulance driving certificates, and later into the IHCD paramedic certificate (Kilner, 2004; Newton, 2012). Staff working for ambulance services had little capacity to influence the outcome of patients and the hospital would have been the only destination for ambulance workers to bring their patients. Today things are very different and continue to change. Some of the drivers for change can be identified as technological advances, raised public expectations of ambulance workers, the establishment of professional and registrant bodies, and legal reform of the National Health Service impacting on the commissioning of healthcare services (DoH, 2013). The second major change in paramedic education came with a move into higher education when the efficacy of the IHCD programme was questioned (Brady, 2014). Initially a very small number of universities in England designed and delivered a paramedic curriculum up to certificate, diploma and degree levels but this increased in line with the Bradley report's call for more appropriate education to support clinical decision making for some 90% of callers not presenting with a life-threatening emergency (DoH, 2005). The shift to higher education has enhanced the attributes, knowledge and skills possessed by paramedics in the modern health economy (Kilner, 2004) and continues to do so as they diversify into wider sectors of healthcare (College of Paramedics, 2017).

The move away from protocol and towards guidelines in paramedic education has enabled paramedics to apply knowledge in a more patient-centred way. There is now a need for paramedics, as well as patients, families and care givers, to have greater knowledge and understanding of what to expect when managing palliative care patients, and patients at the end of their life. Currently there is limited research in this area and much more is needed to generate debate and inform education needs.

Research by Waldrop et al. (2015) identified and discussed four themes highlighted by emergency workers in their assessment and management of patients at the end of their life. These were:

- The undertaking of a multifocal assessment
- The influence of family responses on decision making
- Conflicts of interest among family members
- The management of the dying, including family-witnessed resuscitation and transportation to hospital.

The number of issues for simultaneous and swift assessment is indicative of the level of complexity involved for attending paramedics who, as the title of the article suggests, walk like strangers into someone's life-changing event (Waldrop et al., 2015). The research found that if family dynamics were too conflicting, it was at times easier for emergency workers to take the patient to the emergency department.

One recurring theme in the limited research available is that of paramedics' uncertainty. Studies from the United Kingdom (Murphy-Jones and Timmons, 2016), United States (Stone et al., 2009), Germany (Taghavi et al., 2012; Weise et al., 2012) and Australia (Rogers et al., 2015) have all pointed to anxiety among paramedics concerning their confidence and certainty in decision making at the end of a patient's life. Some sources utilised only small sample sizes from which to draw this observation; however, the larger scale studies concur and all point to a need for educational development in this area. In contrast, research by Waldrop et al. (2014) found a high level of personal confidence among emergency workers, yet even these requested more formal training to specifically manage the legal considerations when utilising and interpreting advance directives.

Appreciation of the traumatic nature of waiting for someone to die may form one aspect of this education with paramedics educated to appreciate the emotional needs of those who make emergency calls. To do this effectively paramedic education may have to include the development of personal emotional awareness training for students. Developing educational needs for paramedic students should also include preparation for dealing with the intensity of family reactions to death through the provision of relevant placement experiences. Enhanced communication skills are needed to confidently and compassionately discuss the fact of actual or imminent death, and these can be built into learning outcomes for student paramedics. JRCALC guidelines on end of life care recognise the distress placed upon care givers at the end of life and recommend debriefing and easy access to staff wellbeing services (JRCALC, 2019).

Formally, the Quality Assurance Agency's (QAA) subject benchmark statements for paramedics state that paramedic education should increase the emphasis on enhanced patient assessment, and on multiprofessional, interdisciplinary practice, to ensure a comprehensive approach to patient care and that the right decision is made at the right time. It states that there should be an 'enhanced focus on reflective, evidence-based practice, to ensure a critical approach to practice and the recognition of the need for continuous quality improvement in the delivery of safe, person centred care' (QAA, 2016: 6). Further to this, the College of Paramedics provide curriculum guidance on dealing with death, bereavement and end of life care (College of Paramedics, 2017). The document includes the study of theories relating to loss and bereavement, the practical knowledge and skills around the use of anticipatory medicines, the recognition of imminent death and administration of supportive care for patients and families. It covers legal and ethical approaches to advance care planning, holistic approach to assessment and management, and forward planning and safety netting.

Organisationally there has been a drive for more locally coordinated end of life care decision-making strategies since the introduction of the *Health and Social Care Act* (DoH, 2012). The result has been the development of Trust responses and continuous professional development learning packages delivered either face to face or online. Finally, recommendations from Waldrop et al. (2014) suggest that, as well as emergency care workers, families, carers and indeed the public would benefit from education regarding the management of expectations at the end of life, and that increasing the knowledge base of other healthcare professionals about the role of out-of-hospital emergency care workers and their scope of practice could also counter misunderstanding.

The Way Forward for Paramedics in the Care of Palliative and End of Life Patients

The research in the previous section points to a desire by participants for greater certainty for patients and their carers and for themselves as attending clinicians. Paramedics identified the need for clearer communication, earlier decision making, and advance planning recorded in an unambiguous manner to facilitate decision making and to ensure the patient's best interests are maintained. Patient-held records have been suggested as a way forward to address these needs (Blackmore, 2016). They are the manifestation of advance care planning, which has been called for by government in the United Kingdom since the *End of Life Care Strategy* (DoH, 2008). In Blackmore's study there was a positive reception for the use of patient-held records from doctors and senior nurses who, like paramedics in previous studies, expressed anxiety and a reduction of professional achievement when they felt that they were not 'getting it right'. As well as assisting the paramedic with decision making, detailed information recorded in patient-held records also prevents unnecessary investigations being undertaken by doctors and nurses in hospital, and prevents patients having to repeat their wishes every time they are seen by a health professional. Problems encountered in previous studies cited by Blackmore indicated concerns regarding the use of patient-held records. These included increasing the workload/burden on the patient, who may not be up to specifying wishes for the end of their life; the risk of breaching patient confidentiality if advance plans were seen inappropriately by family members; and of different services accessing varying computer systems. The latter issue has been addressed by the London-based care plan for integrated urgent care known as 'Coordinate My Care', an information-sharing service providing wraparound access to patients' information regarding management of existing conditions, medications and preferences (Coordinate My Care, 2017). Paramedics can access the Coordinate My Care database via their emergency operations centre either before arrival or at the first opportunity while on scene with the patient.

Paramedics need to have the sophistication in their assessment and management skills to recognise reversible palliative emergencies, other medical emergencies, symptoms associated with stages of deterioration, and the end of life stage. With their greater knowledge and understanding of the principles of palliative care paramedics may initiate discussions with patients and their carers about establishing desires and requirements for latter stages. In this way paramedics may play their role as public educators to provide some structure to their consultation, manage expectations and to establish the goals of care. While the lack of an established therapeutic relationship may be considered a barrier to communication, on the other hand it may provide a refreshing opportunity for patients and their families and carers. Planning for a deterioration before it happens returns control to the patient and opens communication channels with those involved in care giving, where real trust can be established. Where a patient has been able to identify what happens next, which family members/friends should be called, what spiritual support should be in place, what favourite things to be surrounded by, preferred drug and route for analgesia, all contributes to patient-centred care. This also has the benefit of providing some task focus for the attending paramedic, who can have a positive effect on family or carers by enabling the grieving process.

References

Blackmore T (2016). What do acute hospital clinicians think of patient-held records for palliative patients? *European Journal of Palliative Care*, 23(3): 118–123.

Brady M (2012). The concept of a 'good death' in pre-hospital care. *Journal of Paramedic Practice*, 4(12): 688–689.

Brady M (2014). Challenges UK paramedics currently face in providing fully effective end-of-life care. *International Journal of Palliative Nursing*, 20(1): 37–44.

Brown S et al. (2016). *UK Ambulance Services Clinical Practice Guidelines 2016*. Bridgewater: Class Professional Publishing.

College of Paramedics (2017). *Paramedic Curriculum Guidance Handbook* (4th ed.). Bridgewater: College of Paramedics.

Coordinate My Care (2017). *Coordinate My Care, Urgent Care Plan*. Available at: http://coordinatemycare.co.uk/.

Cork A and Brady M (2019). Theories of decision making. In: Blaber A (ed.) *Blaber's Foundations for Paramedic Practice. A Theoretical Perspective* (3rd ed.). New York: McGraw-Hill Education.

Department of Health (2005). *Taking Healthcare to the Patient. Transforming NHS Ambulance Services*. London: Department of Health.

Department of Health (2008). *End of Life Care Strategy – Promoting High Quality Care for all Adults at the End of Life*. London: Department of Health. Available at: https://www.gov.uk/government/publications/end-of-life-care-strategy-promoting-high-quality-care-for-adults-at-the-end-of-their-life.

Department of Health (2012). *Health and Social Care Act*. Available at: http://www.legislation.gov.uk/ukpga/2012/7/contents/enacted/data.htm.

Department of Health (2013). *Paramedic Evidence Based Education Project (PEEP) End of Study Report*. London: Department of Health.

Department of Health (2015). *Policy Paper: 2010 to 2015 Government Policy: Long Term Health Conditions*. London: Department of Health. Available at: http://gov.uk/government/publications/2010-to-2015-government-policy-long-term-health-conditions/2010-to-2015-government-policy-long-term-health-conditions.

Health and Care Professions Council (2016). *Standards of Conduct, Performance and Ethics*. London: Health and Care Professions Council.

JRCALC and AACE (2019). *JRCALC Clinical Guidelines 2019*. Bridgwater: Class Professional Publishing.

Kilner T (2004). Desirable attributes of the ambulance technician, paramedic, and clinical supervisor: findings from a Delphi study. *Emergency Medical Journal*, 21: 374–378.

Murphy-Jones G and Timmons S (2016). Paramedics' experiences of end of life decision making with regard to nursing home residents: an exploration of influential issues and factors. In *Emergency Medical Journal*, 33(10): 722–726.

Newton A (2012). The Ambulance Service: the past, present and future. *Journal of Paramedic Practice*, 4(5): 303–305.

O'Connor S (2018). *Hospice and Palliative Care*. New York: Routledge.

Pope T (2012). How personalised patient care can improve nurses' attitudes to hospitalised older patients. *Nursing Older People*, 24(1): 32–36.

Quality Assurance Agency (2016). *Subject Benchmark Statements Paramedics*. Quality Assurance Agency. Available at: http://dera.ioe.ac.uk/27035/1/SBS-Paramedics-16.pdf.

Rogers I et al. (2015). Paramedics' perceptions and educational needs with respect to palliative care. *Australasian Journal of Paramedicine*, 12(5): 1–7.

Stone S et al. (2009). Paramedic knowledge, attitudes and training in end of life care. *Prehospital and Disaster Medicine*, 24(6): 529–534.

Taghavi M et al. (2012) Paramedics experiences and expectations concerning advance directives: a prospective, questionnaire-based, bi-centre study. *Palliative Medicine*, 26(7): 908–916.

The Kings Fund (2017). *Long-Term Conditions and Multi-Morbidity*. The Kings Fund. Available at: https://www.kingsfund.org.uk/projects/time-think-differently/trends-disease-and-disability-long-term-conditions-multi-morbidity.

Waldrop DP et al. (2014). Preparation for frontline end-of-life care: exploring the perspectives of paramedics and emergency medical technicians. *Journal of Palliative Medicine*, 1(7): 3.

Waldrop DP et al. (2015). 'We are strangers walking into their life-changing event': how prehospital providers manage emergency calls at the end of life. *Journal of Pain and Symptom Management*, 50(3): 328–334.

Wiese C et al. (2012). Paramedics' end of life decision making in palliative emergencies. *Journal of Paramedic Practice*, 4(7): 413–419.

Index

Page numbers followed by *f*, *t* and *b* indicate figures, tables and boxes, respectively.